THE OFFICIAL

DOCTOR/PATIENT

HANDBOOK

A <u>Consumer's</u> Guide
to the
Medical Profession

by
John R.A. Duckworth
Cartoons by Jonathan Pugh

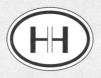

A HARRIMAN HOUSE BOOK

HARRIMAN HOUSE PUBLISHING

'THE OFFICIAL DOCTOR/PATIENT HANDBOOK'

by John R.A. Duckworth

Cartoons by Jonathan Pugh

7 The Spain
Petersfield
Hampshire
GU32 3JZ

Tel. 01730 233870
Fax. 01730 233880

British Library Cataloguing-in-Publication Data

A CIP record for this book is available from the British Library.

ISBN 1 897597 07 X

Printed and bound in Great Britain by

Holbrook Printers Ltd
Norway Rd
Hilsea
Portsmouth
Hants
PO3 5HX

CONTENTS

John Duckworth was born in Lancashire, educated in Yorkshire, and then escaped to the south to read law at Oxford and medicine at a famous London teaching hospital. He is married with four children. He still lives in London where he fantasises about escaping back up north.

PREFACE

Shortly after he had died George was relieved to find himself standing at the Pearly Gates. St. Peter and his staff were busy at the check-in but progress was slow and the queue seemed to stretch for miles.

A group of implausibly attractive girls in white uniforms greeted the new arrivals. One of them approached George, took his arm and escorted him all the way to the back of the queue. As they walked she smiled frequently but did not speak.

"It's busy up here," he said nervously, trying to make conversation.

"You should see the other place," she replied. "Make sure you have your credentials ready for St. Peter."

George took his place. "What credentials?" he thought, and started to worry. It was stiflingly hot and the queue moved slowly. After a few hours an elderly man in front of him was overcome by the heat and fainted. As he fell to the ground, George moved forward to help but before he could do anything there was a thunderclap and a flash of golden light. A figure, clad in white, indistinct and blurred, raced out of the Pearly Gates, picked up the elderly man, and almost instantaneously vanished back into Heaven.

A ripple of conversation spread down the queue. George was frightened. "What was that?" he asked one of the attendants.

"Oh, don't worry," she replied. "That's just God. He likes to play doctor sometimes."

INTRODUCTION

"Physicians of all men are most happy; what good success soever they have, the world proclaimeth, and what faults they commit, the earth coverest."

FRANCIS QUARLES (1592-1644)

• You can survive most illnesses, but can you survive your doctor?

> ➤   How do you know if your doctor is competent?
> ➤   How did he get where he is?
> ➤   Does he tell the truth?
> ➤   Would you know if he doesn't?

This is a book for patients. All patients are people. All people will at some time be patients. Even doctors become patients, although they are not very good at it.

Doctors in particular should read this book. Once upon a time they were people themselves. Some still are. Those that are will enjoy the book. Those that are not will be angry. Or at least they would be if they read it. Probably they will not. So no harm done; no offence caused.

******

• Doctors have traditionally behaved like gods

Secure in the belief that they and only they know what is best for the patient, doctors have felt it neither necessary nor desirable to provide patients with explanations.

Medicine has always been taught on an apprenticeship basis and just as knowledge has been passed down successive generations of doctors, so has prejudice and professional arrogance.

Such a system can have survived only with the tacit consent of the patients. In years gone by they have perceived their doctors to be gods and tolerated, indeed welcomed, high-handed, autocratic treatment. The patient-doctor relationship has been that of parent-child.

The patient as a 'child' has obtained comfort and security from the relationship, but not knowledge. Now the child has come of age. Questions are being asked. Attitudes and manners that have been accepted for years are being scrutinised.

If the child has changed, what about the parent, or doctor? Can he cope with the new relationship? Is the Emperor feeling cold without his clothes?

The *Official Doctor/Patient Handbook* will explain what sort of people become doctors – whether consultants and GPs – how they got where they are, and why they behave as they do.

******

• How rich are doctors?

It is common knowledge that doctors in the United States can earn millions of dollars a year. Can it happen in this country? For the lucky few it can. But which ones? British doctors do not talk about money; or only with each other. Outside the confines of their own profession they adopt the self-righteous stance that money is really rather vulgar.

Few patients even consider how much their doctor earns. There is a general perception that British doctors are hard-working and not as well paid as other professionals like lawyers and accountants.

> ➤ Is it true?
> ➤ Which speciality pays best?
> ➤ What do GPs earn?
> ➤ How are they paid?
> ➤ Are they really overworked?

The *ODPH* reveals all.

• You probably hate going to the doctor.

Most people do. You take every precaution to avoid it. You live your life sensibly and to the full: a healthy diet; plenty of exercise; no tobacco; alcohol in moderation. If, notwithstanding this odd behaviour, you survive to a ripe old age without illness you may think you have permanently escaped the clutches of the medical profession.

But you have not.

Doctors have the ultimate restrictive practice, much envied by lawyers. **You are not allowed to die unless you have communicated your intention, and given valid reasons, to a doctor.**

Perhaps you have managed to get through life without a single medical consultation. Perhaps you have seen a doctor only for trivial matters but have still managed to die without giving due notice or valid reason (In this context advanced old age is not a valid reason). You may think you have escaped and that you can present your body to your Maker unsullied by the medical profession.

Sorry, but you will have to see a doctor after death. He is called a pathologist. You will not be able to choose him and you cannot go privately. Well, you probably could by leaving special instructions in your Will, but your private health insurance will not cover it; and at that stage, who cares?

You would if you knew what really goes on.

The pathologist will cut up your body into little pieces. He will then be able to tell other doctors from which disease you died. If any of the pieces interests him he will keep them for his collection. When he has finished with you, he will return a selection of pieces, many of which will be yours, to your family for disposal.

If you want to be cremated rather than buried, you will have to see *two* doctors. Most people think this is because it is a good idea to have two doctors check that you are really dead if you are going to be burnt. Not true. If you are going to attend your own funeral earlier than strictly necessary, cremation is preferable to burial. Think about it.

No, the need for two doctors to certify death before cremation is down to the lawyers. Lawyers do not like disposing of evidence. Ever. It destroys a potential source of fee generation. Also, lawyers adore second opinions. Why pay one professional to do a job when you can pay two to do it just as badly? If you are buried and a question of foul play arises, they can dig you up for another look. If you have been cremated, well ... that's it. But not if two doctors have certified death. They may disagree. They *will* disagree after they have taken legal advice! More fees.

Thus, whatever strategy you adopt, there can be no escape from the medical profession. You are going to have to go to a doctor at some time. Do not wait until you are dead. Choose one now.

The *ODPH* tells you how to do it.

******

• Sexing the doctor

Throughout this book we shall, unless a specific context warrants otherwise, be referring to doctors as "he". It is of course a common convention to state that "he" encompasses "she". It avoids repeated use of ungainly expressions such as "he or she" or "he/she".

In this book, although "he" may sometimes include "she" it would be grossly misleading, verging on dishonest, to use the convention if it were taken to mean that there are an equal number of male and female practising doctors, or an equality of opportunity for women within the profession.

On the contrary. It was well into the twentieth century before the concept of "female doctor" was viewed as anything other than an oxymoron. To some it is still. The few women that managed to scrape into medical school were overtly and covertly discouraged from any recognised medical career.

Even now, when the intake into medical schools is truly non-sexist (some medical schools take more women than men), the postgraduate training hierarchy has been custom-designed to discriminate against women.

Few women will reach consultant status in the mainstream specialities and those that do are unlikely to be married with children and a normal family life.

- **How doctors relate to you**

Doctors have no training in inter-personal relationships. They learn as they go on.

Or some do.

As they grow older they become increasingly idiosyncratic. They are prone to temper and easily annoyed. Unless you are paying for a private consultation, they have only the convention of good manners to make them polite. Many of them do not feel bound by this convention.

Even now, when the doctor-patient relationship takes place on an adult-adult basis rather than adult-child, it can be difficult to extract the information you require.

What gets up your doctor's nose? Well, you do unless you behave in a certain fashion.

The *ODPH* will show you how to communicate with your doctor in terms he will understand.

******

- **So *you* want to be a doctor?**

The *ODPH* is of particular importance to those people, usually young, who intend to become doctors. By the time you have finished reading you may have changed your mind and decided to be a lawyer; or an architect; in fact, anything but a doctor.

If, however, you are still hanging on in there thinking that medicine is for you, the *ODPH* will show you how to get *into* medical school; how to get *out of it* with a medical qualification and a functioning liver; and which speciality to choose. Above all, it will show you how to climb the postgraduate medical career hierarchy.

Finally, it will teach you how to keep your sanity by retaining insight into your affliction.

The affliction of being 'a doctor'.

******

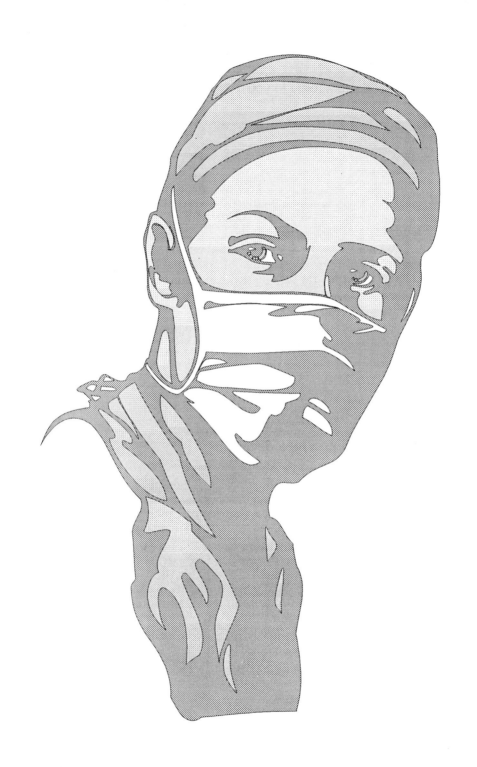

DOCTOR WHO?

What kind of person becomes a doctor?

Deep down, everyone wants to be a doctor. The desire comes on usually at the age of two, sometimes even earlier. Toddlers learn first to play 'Mummies and Daddies' and then graduate to 'Doctors and Patients'. The games are similar in nature. They both involve the swift and unceremonial removal of clothes followed by the exercise of power over another's body. For most children this is a phase, soon outgrown when the attractions of train driving supervene. Those who do not outgrow it go to medical school.

It's a funny business, becoming a doctor. It changes your status. It gives you a title. A title that is held in great respect. If you qualify as an architect or a lawyer, no-one outside the confines of your working life need ever know. You do not book a table at a restaurant in the name of *Architect* Smith; or theatre tickets for *Barrister* Jones. But once you attach the magic word 'Doctor' to your name, you are perceived differently. Doors open.

Why is this? Because people are frightened of doctors. A doctor knows more about their bodies than they know themselves. Therefore he has power over them.

We should *all* become doctors then no-one would be afraid of them.

So why *don't* we all become doctors? Many reasons, not least the hard work involved. For the would-be doctor, there is tiresome legislation in this country requiring those wishing to practise medicine to attend medical school and obtain a recognised qualification in medicine; or to be more precise, a qualification in *medicine, surgery and midwifery*.

There is some logic to this requirement: it protects people from unprincipled charlatans. In the old days, anyone could offer medical treatment, including surgery, to the great general public. And many did. The doctors regarded surgery as unnecessary, poorly paid and, worst of all, messy. Surgery was therefore performed by the barbers whose shops were marked with the famous red and white pole. Doctors would have nothing to do with the barber-surgeons and in particular would not allow them to style themselves as 'Doctor'. They had to remain plain 'Mr'.

When surgery was finally recognised by Parliament and incorporated within the medical Acts, the surgeons, as a sort of inverted snobbery, continued to refer to themselves as 'Mr'.

Of course anyone can still practise medicine, and many do. They are the 'alternative' practitioners. Not allowed by law to call themselves 'Doctor' they practise a variety of trades from the ridiculous to the sublime. Many are competent. A few are not. As a rule of thumb their ability is inversely proportional to the number of letters they have after their name.

You cannot obtain a real medical degree by correspondence course nor by distance learning. There is as yet no Open University degree in medicine. The only way to become a doctor is by demonstrating your ability and suitability to enter a recognised medical school.

The public is thus protected.

Or is it?

Who is deemed 'suitable' to enter medical school? Those who are able may not be suitable, and vice versa. The traditionalists in the medical profession whole-heartedly support a highly selective and discriminatory entry into the profession. Not to protect the general public though. The real purpose is to protect themselves from an influx of undesirables.

They are not prepared to tolerate any old Tom, Dick or Harry - and certainly not any old Wayne, Shane, Abdul, Asif, Charlotte, Jane or Tracy - putting a plate up outside their house and calling themselves 'Doctor'.

Who then is most likely to go to medical school? How should the would-be medical student prepare himself?

Entry into Medical School

Competition for medical school places is fierce. There are as many as twenty applicants for each place. Most will have A-levels in Physics, Chemistry and Biology and so will have specialised in scientific disciplines from the age of fifteen or sixteen.

Until ten years ago a few medical schools ran a pre-medical year (called 1st MB) which allowed entry to medical school for those with arts A-levels or even arts graduates. No more.

The medical schools are so spoilt for choice that getting three A grades is no guarantee of a place. Many highly qualified applicants will be disappointed.

Should your doctor be a doctor?

All medical exams, from the basic first qualification at medical school, to the highest-of-the-high specialist exams have a failure rate.

There is indeed an honourable tradition of having many attempts to pass professional exams at all levels. Marks are never made public. A pass or a fail is awarded. A handful of candidates may get 'Honours' or 'Gold Medals'. Some pass easily. Others only scrape through. The public never knows which doctors only just made it.

This gives rise to the engaging proposition that, scattered through the country, in each area of expertise, there must a group of doctors who were borderline. The man about to take out your appendix may have became a surgeon only at the twenty-third attempt, and then by half of one per cent.

If we accept the validity of exams as predictors of medical ability - and that itself is a vexed issue - we must also accept that we can on objective criteria identify the worst doctor in the country. Do his patients know who he is? Does he know? He might be your doctor.

Of course, grading doctors is not as easy as that. Practical experience counts for much. The ability to communicate humanely with patients - a skill traditionally ignored or even derided at the older medical schools - is paramount.

The *ODPH* will help you decide if your doctor is competent.

Would *you* make a good doctor?

Perhaps you are thinking of a career in medicine.

Think hard.

Before you expose yourself to the trauma of rejection, are you sure you really want to be a doctor? Could you survive the training? Are you suitable material?

British medical schools have been secretive to the point of paranoia about their real entry criteria. Good science A-levels are only the starting point. Background, school, social class, nationality, parents' occupation, sex and many other factors are taken into account.

What makes a doctor can best be summed up in one word: ATTITUDE. Exam results and background help, but what really governs a student's ability to get in and out of medical school is his willingness to take on the culture and ethos of the medical establishment. What is his attitude to patients? To illness? To colleagues? Does he have, or can he acquire, *medical machismo*?

What is medical machismo?

No-one will tell you. It is often congenital but may be acquired. It can certainly be nurtured. Medical schools believe that the best way to measure a doctor's competence is by making him take multiple choice examinations (MCQs). The following is an example of the sort of MCQ medical students take. This one has been designed to measure **your** medical machismo. It will also accurately predict:

> ➢ The likelihood of you being accepted by a medical school.
>
> ➢ The career path you should take in medicine.
>
> ➢ The kind of doctor you will be.
>
> ➢ Your likely level of success.

Those *not* wishing to be doctors - the majority of you - should take the test anyway. It will give you an insight into the value of these splendid examinations.

The Medical Machismo Test

The following MCQ should be completed within fifteen minutes. Tick the answers you think are correct. More than one answer may be correct in each question. Leave the others blank. Go on your gut feeling. It rarely helps to think.

1. **To the best of your knowledge are you:**

   (a) Male

   (b) Female

   (c) Indeterminate

   (d) All of the above

   (e) It depends who is asking

2. **The careers master asks if you prefer round or oval balls. Do you:**

   (a) Giggle

   (b) Goose him

   (c) Invite him round for dinner when your parents are out

   (d) Start singing 'Land of my fathers'

   (e) Phone Esther Rantzen

3. **Your little sister runs into your room crying because her goldfish has stopped swimming and sunk to the bottom of the bowl. Would you:**

   (a) Flush it down the lavatory

   (b) Put some brandy in the bowl

   (c) Cut it up with your penknife to see if it is dead

   (d) Ask if it has private insurance

   (e) Deep fry it for supper

4. **Was "The Lady with the Lamp":**
   (a) A transexual coalminer
   (b) A man-servant
   (c) A health care pioneer
   (d) A sexual facilitator for doctors
   (e) Dixon of Dock Green's wife

5. **Where were you educated?**
   (a) A famous public school
   (b) A state school
   (c) A single sex-school
   (d) A co-ed school
   (e) Wot, like . . . er, exams an that?

6. **You are a doctor. You are on a cross-channel ferry when a passenger jumps overboard. An announcement is made asking for a doctor to come forward. Would you:**
   (a) Run to the bridge to offer help
   (b) Walk to the bridge to offer help
   (c) Hide in the lavatory
   (d) Go and buy your Duty Free
   (e) Miss the message because you have already drunk your Duty Free and are comatose

7. **Amongst your relatives there are (is) :**
   (a) Two or more consultant surgeons
   (b) An eminent female physician
   (c) At least one GP
   (d) A hospital cleaner or a practising psychiatrist
   (e) An England cap in rugby or cricket (*not* soccer or darts)

14

8. Do you think that doctors are:

(a) On average better paid than lawyers

(b) More trustworthy than politicians

(c) Good lovers

(d) More useful than undertakers

(e) Well-educated

9. What is you worst fault? (Be honest)

(a) Sexism

(b) Racial prejudice

(c) Elitism

(d) All of the above and more

(e) Difficult to think of any worth mentioning

10. 'Nurses are sexy.' What is your reaction to this assertion?

(a) Typical oppressive heterosexist stereotype.

(b) Even Robin Cook would look sexy in a nurse's uniform.

(c) It's a mother/whore thing.

(d) Not when they're giving you an enema, they're not.

(e) In American sitcoms maybe, in reality never.

11. What is the primary advantage of mother's milk over powdered milk?

(a) It has all the nutrients needed to sustain a baby

(b) It is protected from germs and infection by the mother.

(c) It is always served at the right temperature.

(d) It comes in such nice containers.

(e) Powdered milk is a cynical tool of capitalist empire-building.

12. **Which of the following do you think would be most helpful in achieving a successful medical career:**

    (a) An interest in human biology

    (b) A desire to help people

    (c) A repertoire of funny handshakes

    (d) Oval balls

    (e) A brace of godparents on the interviewing panel

13. **How soon after child birth is it reasonable to expect a woman to resume sexual intercourse?**

    (a) About six weeks

    (b) As soon as she feels like it

    (c) As soon as her husband feels like it, but a gentleman waits until the placenta has been delivered

    (d) Intercourse is only allowed with the doctor's permission

    (e) Intercourse is only allowed with the doctor

14. **British medical students are characteristically:**

    (a) Hard-working

    (b) Interested in the arts

    (c) Against pre-marital sex

    (d) Working class idealists

    (e) Drunk

15. **When the Israeli medical profession went on strike, the national death rate fell.This demonstrates that:**

    (a) Statistics are meaningless

    (b) Jewish doctors are anti-Semitic

    (c) Euthanasia should be illegal.

    (d) Robert Maxwell may still be alive

    (e) Israel is a far away country of which we know nothing.

NOW CHECK YOUR SCORE

1. Deduct 20 marks if the questionnaire took more than 15 minutes.

2. Add up your marks using the grid below. (Note that some answers attract *minus* marks)

3. Read off your personal evaluation below.

Question	(a)	(b)	(c)	(d)	(e)
1	10	2	5	7	15
2	12	4	2	1	7
3	8	3	6	10	1
4	1	4	0	10	4
5	10	0	8	2	6
6	0	4	2	10	8
7	10	2	3	0	-5
8	8	2	10	1	15
9	8	8	8	10	15
10	0	3	2	- 5	10
11	4	5	5	15	8
12	2	0	8	10	3
13	5	3	1	10	5
14	0	0	0	0	5
15	8	2	9	10	3

Personal Evaluation

Those of you scoring between 50 and 199 marks can expect to be doctors of one sort or another. You will be sub-categorised into one of four groups depending upon your mark. Rupert, Georgina, James and Kevin will be a typical member of each group, and their subsequent careers will be followed throughout the book. Of course, one or more of Rupert, James and Kevin is or are likely to be female. We have deliberately upset the balance to provoke female readers who have ambitions to go into medicine. If overt sexism of this sort offends you, be a nurse. You will not survive in medicine.

Over 200
This score is not possible. You have been cheating and, worse still, you have been caught. Such effrontery has no place in the medical profession. Be a lawyer.

150 - 199
Congratulations! Very encouraging. Arrogance tempered with insensitivity. You may already be a doctor. If not, daddy must be. You are prejudiced, self-opinionated and intolerant. You will not let human frailty, pain or suffering deflect you from your objectives. Go straight to medical school. Consider surgery. A career in a London Teaching Hospital is likely. (RUPERT)

100 - 149
Much promise here. Females scoring in this range are the equivalent of males in the 150 - 200 range. They will find it tough in London but may make it in the provinces. Consider general medicine. (GEORGINA)

50 - 99
Well, anything is possible but it will be difficult for you to succeed in hospital medicine. You show a complete lack of arrogance, an ability to get on with people, and humility. Consider general practice. (JAMES)

0 - 49
Are you sure you really want to be a doctor? If so, your only hope is psychiatry. Possibly community medicine. Good luck. You will need it. (KEVIN)

Minus scores
No, no, no. Completely hopeless. You are looking at the wrong career. Consider one of the caring professions.

How Medical Schools Select Students

"I believe, indeed, that fifty years ago the admission of young ladies to be nurses in this [Bart's] or any similar hospital could not have been seriously proposed. It would have been called indecent, audacious, unprincipled, and I know not what besides; and the notion of their being associated with medical students would have been deemed utterly vile; nothing but vile mischief would have been foretold of it."

SIR JAMES PAGET (1814-99)

Ability or Suitability?

By now, you will be beginning to get an idea of the qualities required for a successful career in medicine. If you scored well in the Medical Machismo Test you may even be considering going to medical school yourself. We shall now look in detail at the peculiar mix of ability and suitability that, when filtered through the prejudicial admissions procedure, will guarantee a place at medical school. The characteristics of the candidate traditionally most likely to get into medical school appear in the table below.

In years gone by, these qualifications alone would guarantee a place at medical school. If an interview was felt to be necessary at all, it would consist of a friendly chat with the Dean who would enquire after father and reminisce about the rugby they used to play together. The place would

The traditional medical student

Gender	Male
Family Socio-Economic Group	Professional/Managerial
Father/Mother's Job	Doctor
Class	Middle, wealthy middle
School	Public, single-sex
Sporting Achievements and other	Considerable, often rugby or rowing
A-levels	Three A grades or close
Age of Entry	17 or 18 – straight from school

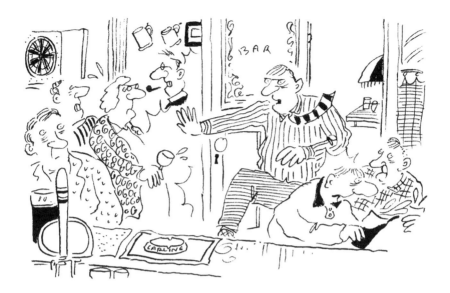

"Let me through, I'm a doctor"

be confirmed shortly afterwards.

And so, if you went to any British medical school in the first week of the Autumn term to meet the archetypal tyro medical student, what did you find?

A recently pubescent eighteen year old rugger-bugger, who we shall call Rupert.

Rupert's experience of life has been provided exclusively within the confines of his all-male public school. If it is after five o'clock he will have a pint of beer in his hand. He will tell you that daddy was at the same medical school in the early 1960s and that his record for the Yard of Ale Projectile Vomit Competition still stands at eighteen feet.

He thinks he is well-educated because his public school has crammed three good science A-Levels into him. He has never read any literature. Ask him if he would like a book for his birthday and he will decline saying he has already got one; and that will be by Jeffrey Archer.

He has a student nurse on his arm who he does not introduce because he has forgotten her name but he will tell you in a loud stage whisper that later he is going to "shag the arse off her".

Go back at ten o' clock. The nurse has long since disappeared, bored to tears. Rupert is still going strong. He may or may not have his trousers on, but either way is making valiant attempts to break daddy's record, surrounded by friends singing songs about Indian Warriors.

Is it still like this?

No.

Or not entirely. There is still a large contingent of Ruperts at medical school, and their curriculum vitae remain highly marketable. But there has been a major change, or widening, in entry criteria. Georgina, James and Kevin are there as well. Georgina is rarely in the bar. She is more likely to be in the library. She is frightened by Rupert. James and Kevin are not afraid of him; they hold him in contempt. They do not take off their trousers when they are drinking beer.

The move away from a legion of Ruperts has been brought about by medical schools' tardy and grudging recognition of the fact that the medical students they were choosing were the ones least likely to have a successful career in medicine.

As a rough generalisation, the medical student who does best has the following characteristics: she is female, from a lower-middle class, non-medical background; she has been to a state school; she has had a break between school and university, perhaps doing VSO; she has studied another discipline before coming to medicine. She is . . . Georgina

Thirty years ago, if senior schools had not successfully discouraged Georgina, the medical schools, with the exception of the Royal Free, completed the job by refusing entry to all but the most talented; and the definition of 'most talented' would hinge on the interview committee's assessment of whether the woman was likely to give up a career to have children.

This has all gone. Entry is genuinely non-sexist. There remains a strong class bias. There is some racial prejudice. Rupert still stands a better chance than most but he only has a small corner of the student bar now, and his activities are met more with indifference than approbation.

Entry for students with arts A-levels or arts degrees was always taxing as they were faced with the pre-medical 1st MB course, meaning six years at medical school rather than five. Often they would have no entitlement to a grant, or certainly not for the first three years.

The disappearance of 1st MB has made entry for these people even more difficult. Now they may have to do three science A-levels at home.

Having arrived at medical school, the student is insulated from the worst prejudices of the profession for five years. He should be aware though that the respite is only temporary. After qualification, sexism and racial prejudice will again be encountered.

The medical student most likely to succeed

Gender	Female
Family Socio-Economic Group	Blue Collar
Father/Mother's Job	Non-medical, non-professional
Class	Working, lower-middle
School	State school, often co-educational
Sporting Achievements	Not relevant
A-levels	Good – not necessarily the best
Age of Entry	Early twenties

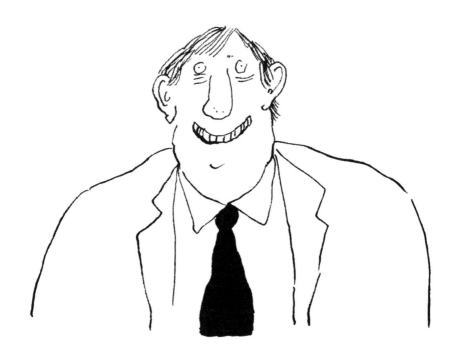

"Six munfs ago, I cudn't even spel docta. Now I are wun."

THE MEDICAL CURRICULUM

"There is no person, let his situation in life be what it may, whom, if I were so disposed to dissect, I could not obtain."

SIR ASTLEY COOPER (1768-1841)
Surgeon to Royalty, explaining to the House of Commons
Committee how he acquired bodies for dissection.

What do doctors learn?

Assuming he passed all his exams first time, your doctor spent five years at medical school. The core of his curriculum has not changed in over a century.

The first two years are spent studying the three basic medical sciences of *anatomy, physiology* and *biochemistry.*

These subjects are intensely boring and of little relevance to the art of practising medicine. They are often badly taught by people who, only sometimes unfairly, are assumed to be failed doctors.

The extraordinary tradition of compelling students to dissect a human body, starting on the first day of their medical careers, persists. All medical students are nervous as they approach the dissection room to meet their first patient. These are the only patients they will have in their careers who have died *before* they have met them. It is also the first and only time that they are not likely to be sued for any mistakes. And just as well. Few parents would allow their seventeen-year old son or daughter to carve the Sunday roast. Why should they do any better with a human body? They do not.

They learn to call their first patient a cadaver. This is a euphemism for "dead body". Human dissection is a rite of passage. It is about machismo. Rupert is the one most likely to faint. Georgina loves it. James and Kevin put up with it. All four of our heroes begin to develop a 'medical' sense of humour in the dissection room.

At the end of two years, students take an exam in the basic sciences and if successful will be allowed to progress to the three clinical years during which they are exposed to patients. Or more correctly, patients are exposed to them. Literally and metaphorically. The word clinical has connotations of precise scientific research and study. In fact, it comes from a Greek word meaning "bedside". And that is where the clinical medical student learns – at the patient's bedside.

There have been some improvements in medical education this century. Originally, anatomists had to rely on bribing gravediggers to obtain their supply of dead bodies. This was a nice little earner for the impoverished gravediggers but alas for them the system was nationalised. A reliable source of dead bodies is now provided by HMG. Anyone who feels they have finished with their body may volunteer for dissection by telephoning the London Anatomy Office on 081-981-9390.

Other disciplines have been added to the traditional three. These include, for example, *pharmacology*, which is the study of drugs and what drugs do to patients. More recently, with the realisation that doctors occasionally have to talk to patients, subjects such as *sociology* and *psychology* have appeared. These are trendy subjects. Rupert does not approve and will miss all the lectures pleading rugby practice.

Vague attempts are made to introduce pre-clinical medical students to real patients. Most are risible. A two-hour session is put aside, probably on a Friday afternoon, for such clinical exposure.

In theory an intelligent and willing in-patient happily agrees to see a few junior medical students.

In reality, what happens is something like this. A consultant is stuck in a traffic jam on the way to Harley Street. Suddenly he recalls that he is supposed to be giving a talk to the pre-clinical students. He uses his carphone to contact his registrar and asks him to deputise. The registrar bleeps the houseman and tells him to find a patient. The houseman has not had any lunch; there are three emergencies waiting for him in Casualty and he has just heard that his girlfriend has missed her last period. He rushes to the ward and railroads the first gullible punter he can find into going for a ride in a wheelchair with never a mention of the fact that he is about to be asked to display his scrotal swelling· to a hundred and ten giggly teenagers.

Character building - *laughing at illness, disease and tragedy*

The average British teenager has had no experience of serious illness. He has had no real contact with death. The nearest he has come was as an eight-year old when he used to catch Daddy Long Legs and put them in spiders' webs.

His parents are alive and although he may have lost a grand parent he probably did not go to the funeral. He cannot yet comprehend his own mortality. Death is something that happens to other people; to people he does not know. As a result, he has no idea how to cope with it nor how to cope with the serious illness that may precede it. It may frighten him. It embarrasses him. Subconsciously or semi-subconsciously he knows that it is something that profoundly affects patients and yet he dare not let it affect him. He deals with it inappropriately. He may even snigger. What he must not do is show emotion. That would not be in the finest tradition of medical machismo.

Medical machismo is founded in the dissection room. Walking into a room full of naked dead bodies is a traumatic and unpleasant experience. Didn't old Auntie Ethel leave her body to medical science? Pull back the cover and, Oh God! there she is.

It has happened.

You have to laugh. What else can you do?

Rupert may well have fainted, but after that soon gets into the swing of things. He removes the bones from one of the fingers in his cadaver and inserts them, through a small underside slit, into the penis of Georgina's cadaver.

When she gets to this part of the dissection Rupert and the boys chortle as she flips through the pages of Gray's Anatomy trying to find the penile bone. When she gives up and asks the professor about it they stuff their handkerchiefs in their mouths, helpless with laughter. If the Professor is a Rupert, he leads Georgina further down the garden path. More likely he will tell her not to be so naive and tiresome. Of course, he sees this practical joke every year; he invented it himself as a student.

The first doctor-patient relationship formed in the dissecting room between an immature teenager and a dead body is formative and never forgotten.

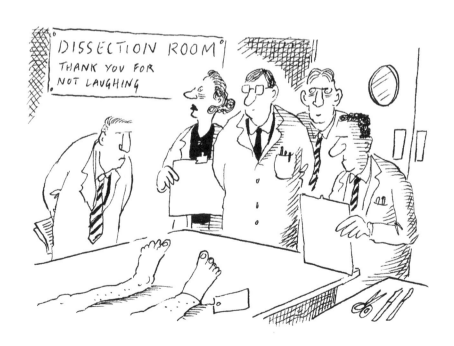

Continual Assessment - *progressive harassment*

Exams are the medical student's constant companion. Traditionally there are two big ones: the exam in basic medical sciences at the end of two years and then finals at the end of the three clinical years.

The bane of the medical student's life is the *viva*. This is the usual method of assessing his progress throughout the undergraduate training and at the final examinations. The stress and fear induced in students by vivas is intense and lays the foundations for the way they will treat colleagues, particularly junior colleagues, in the future.

Imagine making a soufflé from a Delia Smith recipe in front of Delia Smith; or playing the Moonlight Sonata in front of Beethoven. Describing the blood supply to the pancreas to the editor of Gray's Anatomy is equally challenging and not helped by the fact that he is unlikely to be gentle, kind and charming, and is certainly not deaf.

Written exams and vivas occur every three months throughout the medical student's career and are a constant worry. He knows only too well that the penalty for repeated failure is expulsion.

Many examiners specialise in cruelty. Females get a hard time from male examiners and males get a hard time from the increasingly common female examiners.

This climate of fear creates a regime in which knowledge is acquired not through interest in the subject, nor for its own sake, but on pain of death; or worse - ritual humiliation.

The anatomy viva is most frightening of all. The student faces two or more examiners, all eminent in their field. He finds his modest but adequate knowledge is trapped behind tongue-tied fear. He is given no help, no time to gather his thoughts. Soon, the professor interrupts one of his stammering answers:

"Look out of the window, *doctor*. What do you see?"

"Er... er... nothing in particular, sir"

"Trees, *doctor*, trees"

"Yes, sir"

"And what colour are the leaves, *doctor*?"

"Green, sir."

"Well spotted, *doctor*. Come back when they are brown."

And so he departs, only a few minutes into the viva, deprived of the opportunity of redemption, and knowing that the repeat viva in six months time will be his last chance to stay at medical school.

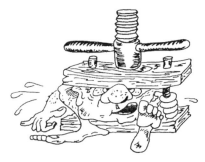

"Go on you bastard, give it another turn! I work better under pressure."

Learning to criticise colleagues

Some medical students repeatedly fail the examinations in basic medical sciences. They are kicked out. One or two realise early on that medicine is not for them and leave of their own volition. The majority (over 95%) pass and thus after two brief years at medical school, at the age of nineteen or twenty, they find themselves on the wards in contact with real patients.

Clinical medical students are still taught as apprentices. They are divided into groups and attached to a particular consultant and his team. The collective noun for a consultant and his team is a "Firm".

Over the three years of their clinical training, students rotate through various firms covering all the major specialist areas of medicine. Thus in theory they receive a broad-based education. But not in practice.

The clinical training period lasts three years but of this, three months will be spent on an elective period of study and a further six months must be allowed for holidays and exams. This leaves twenty-seven months. Each appointment lasts three months, so there is time for nine appointments in total. Four of these will be taken up with the traditional 'mainstream' and 'most important' specialities of *general medicine* and *general surgery*. One will be devoted to *obstetrics & gynaecology*, one to *orthopaedics*, one to *psychiatry*, and one to *paediatrics*. And yet less than twenty per cent of the students will become consultants in all of these specialities put together.

This leaves **one three-month appointment** for the student to learn *anaesthetics, child psychiatry, dermatology, geriatrics, haematology, microbiology, neurology, oncology, ophthalmology, otolaryngology, radiology, radiotherapy, rheumatology, traumatology, urology,* and *venereology*.

It cannot be done.

In order to cover the medical syllabus, these 'minor' specialities are scattered in a random fashion amongst other firms. Inevitably the students regard them as less important subjects. The resulting firms have an incongruous mix of disciplines. One medical school had a triple appointment in *psychiatry, orthopaedics* and *venereology*. 'Nuts, bolts and screws' is how the students termed it. When it was realised that there was too much work in the appointment, and *psychiatry* was re-allocated, the firm became 'dicks and sticks'.

General practice, which is the speciality that most students will enter, may have no definite appointment at all. At best, perhaps a week or two squeezed in between, say, *obstetrics & gynaecology* and *general medicine*.

The consultants in the major specialities resent the students having to devote any of their time to other activities and openly deride the 'minor' specialities and, by implication, their specialists. Try telling a consultant surgeon in a London teaching hospital that you have to leave his operating list to attend a psychiatry tutorial. Rupert would not dream of so doing. He never goes to psychiatric tutorials anyway. Georgina attends all tutorials and so timidly begs leave to go. She pretends not to hear the consultant's contemptuous remarks about being off to "learn from the clever doctors". Kevin has already decided that he wants to be a psychiatrist and so is not at the operating list in the first place. James compromises and alternates between the list and the tutorial. This offends both the surgeon and the psychiatrist who only notice James when he is absent.

Students soon learn a pecking order of the various specialities. Of course, the pecking order varies according to viewpoint. Objectively, it would be difficult to decide whether the psychiatrists treat the surgeons with greater contempt than the surgeons treat the psychiatrists.

The Ward Round:
The Spanish Inquisition

A firm in a provincial district general hospital may well consist only of a consultant and a houseman, being led round the ward by one nurse.

The ward round conducted by a senior consultant surgeon and his firm at a London teaching hospital is much more impressive to behold. Mannerisms and dress alone betray enough psycho-social pathology for a psychiatric thesis.

There is apparent over-manning. Not really, of course, because the consultant is usually in Harley Street and only appears on the NHS wards for one hour a week. Likewise, the senior registrar is usually absent doing research.

Sister leads the way with one of her student nurses pushing the notes trolley. Except for the occasional frosty criticism, Sister ignores the student nurse. She chats to the consultant in an over-friendly manner, sometimes, if she is brave, calling him by his first name. This is to show that she is a fellow professional and a social equal.

The consultant does not wear a white coat because not wearing a white coat is his uniform, his distinguishing mark. He is intensely irritated by what he sees as the inappropriately familiar manner of the Sister, but dare not say anything because, unlike his junior staff who come and go, Sister is one of the fixtures-and-fittings and could make his life hell if he does not co-operate. He affects a matey, conspiratorial and flirty relationship, but behind her back tells friends that he hasn't screwed her because she has an arse the size of Clapham Common.

The senior registrar will be wearing a white coat unless:

1. He thinks he ought to have a consultant appointment.
2. He has a consultant appointment to take up in the near future.
3. He is a pompous shit.
4. All of the above apply.

He chats to the consultant treating him as an equal, although he considers himself intellectually superior. The consultant is charming to the senior registrar, because:

1. He is about to become a consultant colleague and social equal.
2. He looks after the NHS patients enabling the consultant to stay on Harley Street seeing private patients.
3. He is more knowledgeable

The registrar is somewhere in between. He is the workhorse of the firm. He has to stay friendly with the senior registrar because he needs help occasionally and it is not that long ago that he was a house officer so he still has traces of human decency.

The senior house officer (SHO) is smart and alert. He has finished his year as a house officer but has little experience. He is above the scut work but cannot yet do anything useful. He is studying hard for postgraduate exams. He watches the registrar at work and sniggers conspiratorially when the house officer is criticised. In the teaching hospital he is supernumerary.

The house officer is the gopher. He does all the jobs no-one else wants to do. His white coat is creased and dirty. His pockets are bulging with notepads and he tries to hide his constant companion – a well-thumbed copy of 'The I-Spy Book of Operations'. Everyone on the firm shits on him. He has a badge saying, "Don't even ask - it's my fault."

Last of all come the medical students. There may be twelve or more of them. Sparklingly clean white coats, intense faces, pens poised over notebooks. Georgina is at the front, looking receptive. James and Kevin are somewhere in the middle, day-dreaming. Rupert brings up the rear, ogling the student nurses.

The only time the firm comes together with a unity of purpose is in the last ten minutes of the ward round when the boss decides it is "time to teach the boys and girls".

They gather round a patient's bed. The junior doctors melt to the back to gossip quietly with Sister. The medical students are pushed forward. The ritual humiliation begins. They may only have been clinical medical students for a few days. They will have had no guidance on reading. They have no chance of answering the consultant's questions.

The patient selected will have a rare, small-print condition. The boss is sexist and takes particular pleasure in humiliating young girls. He singles out Georgina.

"Take a look at this patient's face. What do you notice?"

"Er... nothing... er... abnormal, sir" she stammers.

The boss glances over to the juniors for a team snigger. Rupert-class students also snigger knowingly although they cannot see anything abnormal either. But the boss is President of the Rugby Club. He will not pick them out.

James and Kevin do not snigger because they are at risk. And indeed it is finally their turn. By a stroke of luck, Kevin happens to remember the obscure medical condition the boss is hinting at, and comes out with the correct answer. The boss pounces:

"Found the library, have you Kevin? Perhaps you'll tell everyone else where it is, there's a good chap."

Kevin is labelled as a brown-nose.

The medical student cannot win. Absence of knowledge results in humiliation; presence of knowledge is ridiculed. But already he is acquiring one new skill. The unnatural art of

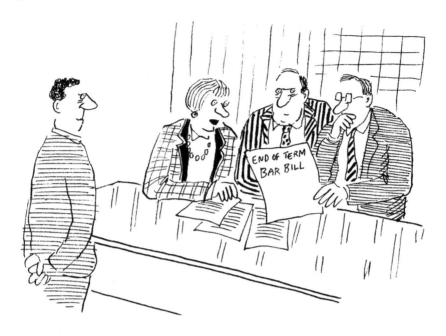

How to Tell if a Doctor is Fit to Practise

taking pleasure from the criticism or even the humiliation of colleagues. Rupert gets there first. The others will soon follow.

Finals - *how to tell if a doctor is fit to practise*

At the end of five years study, two years academic pre-clinical and three years apprenticeship on the wards, medical students take an exam to see if they are fit to become doctors. If they pass the exam they are entitled to put the letter MB BS (MB ChB for northerners and MB BChir for Oxbridge graduates) after their name and call themselves 'Doctor'.

The student has the opportunity to take final medical examinations set by three different organisations.

1. The university he attends;

2. The Conjoint Examiners' Board which is an amalgamation of the Royal Colleges of Surgeons, Physicians and Obstetricians & Gynaecologists;

3. The Society of Apothecaries.

The most sought after is the university qualification, but each and any of them enables the doctor to practise. It is sometimes said that the weakest candidates will take all three to give themselves the best chance of passing. Whilst there is some truth in this, in the main students recognise the huge luck element involved in passing first time. Taking finals from multiple boards is not so much cynicism as a form of sensible insurance.

Final exams are divided into two parts: written and clinical. The clinical part always takes place at a different hospital to the one at which the student trained. The clinical is divided into 'the long case' and 'the short cases.' For the long case, the student will have about forty-five minutes to take a history from a patient and examine him. He presents his findings to the examiner and they discuss how he would manage the problems he has identified.

The examiner then takes him round four or five patients – the short cases – asking him to demonstrate physical examination techniques and quizzing him on the significance of clinical signs.

The patients acting as examination fodder will all have long-standing stable illnesses with obvious physical signs. They are unpaid, but get transport to and from the hospital plus the inevitable free cup of tea and a bun. They love it. They are thoroughly familiar with their illnesses and more clued-up on their physical signs than their doctors. Most of them will give a helping hand to the puzzled and nervous student who has been listening to their heart murmur for ten minutes. "It's mitral stenosis, and there is a loud opening snap. Rheumatic fever, you know." Never offend these patients. They know what the examiners want to hear.

In non-medical university exam papers candidates typically have a choice of questions; they have to answer, say, four out of the ten questions set. Astute candidates look at past papers, work out which subjects always come up, and on that basis, jettison a quarter of the syllabus. This leaves them free to concentrate on the bits they enjoy, and still get first-class honours.

Medical students, who have a vast syllabus to learn, would die for this kind of *laissez-faire* examination policy. Alas, so might the patients entrusted to their care:

> "I'm so sorry, Mrs Arkwright, but I always found heart attacks rather boring at medical school so I missed them out."

Patients will be reassured to know that the examining bodies at medical schools have solved the problem of choice in exams. There is no choice. Nothing is excluded. All parts of the syllabus must be covered in detail.

So thank God for that. Fully-rounded doctors is what we want. Or is it? No choice means lower standards. The medical student who has to cover a huge syllabus may end up knowing nothing about everything. Arguably that is no better than the sociology student who can cherry-pick his syllabus, but who ends up knowing everything about nothing.

What does the basic qualification mean anyway? It certainly doesn't indicate that the holder is going to be a good doctor. It is recognition of the fact that the student has attained the standards required by the examination board and nothing else. You cannot measure a doctor. The final exam is the first entrance exam. It acknowledges the probability that the student is fit to begin real medical training.

The analogy of the driving test is a good one. It is only after you pass your driving test and start driving alone that you really begin to learn how to drive. The newly-qualified doctor is in a similar position. There is however one important difference. The newly-qualified driver is practising on the A35.

The newly-qualified doctor is practising on you.

Acquiring bad habits

"An alcoholic is a man who drinks more than his doctor"

ANON

When it comes to drinking, doctors are in the big league. They are up there with journalists, publicans and the French. The foundations for a lifetime's drinking are laid at medical school and built upon during junior hospital jobs.

Lectures and ward commitments in most medical schools finish at five o'clock in the afternoon, which is when the bar opens. As in all student unions, beer is cheap. Full advantage is taken.

Medical student culture revolves round beer and rugby. Tales of prodigious drinking abound. If the student finds his ability to consume vast quantities of alcohol are flagging, there are numerous songs, well known in the rugby club, to help, and there are even specific drinking games. Let us consider one of the most popular – **'Fourjacks'**.

Equipment required

1. One pack of playing cards

2. At least four players

3. A half-pint beer mug for each player

4. A large bucket

Rules

1. The players sit in a circle.

2. The dealer shuffles the pack and starts dealing, one card to each player.

3. The first player to receive a Jack specifies a particular drink.

4. The second player to receive one buys it.

5. The third takes a sip and describes the drink to the assembled throng.

6. The fourth player downs it in one.

7. Any player vomiting in the bucket has to replenish the drink and do it again.

The concoctions become increasingly absurd and unpleasant. A barley wine with a double amontillado sherry. Sounds innocuous. Try it.

Mind-numbing games such as these are a common way for tomorrow's doctors to idle away their free time. They are accepted, indeed admired, as part of developing medical machismo.

Medical students arriving in the bar at five o'clock consume three or four pints of beer without noticing it. Five or six nights a week. And then there are long evenings after rugby matches when consumption is even higher. Thirty to forty pints a week is commonplace. And quite often it is pints of strong lager, not just ordinary cooking bitter.

Doctors classify alcoholic drink in terms of units.

One unit of alcohol is equal either to half a pint of bitter, a small measure of spirits (i.e. a single pub measure, not the average slosh that is poured at home), a small sherry or a small glass of wine. Thirty pints of beer a week is sixty units.

Rupert manages his sixty units with gusto and aplomb. James and Kevin are well up there. And do not think that Georgina is teetotal. She may seem to drink less than the boys, but alcohol excess is not a male preserve. Georgina has a bottle of Martini in her room 'for emergencies.'

Drinking is rife, recognised and catered for. At one famous London teaching hospital in the seventies the junior hospital doctors' accommodation was being refurbished. The question was whether to authorise the considerable extra expense of putting wash basins in all the rooms. The committee, aware of the beer intake, thought the young doctors would pee in the sinks and so were against it. Then it was pointed out that if there were no sinks, they would pee out of the window. The rooms overlook the consultants' car park. Sinks were installed.

Most student bars in universities throughout the country have an element of serious drinking but why is it so prevalent at medical schools? Because it answers the need for an instant release of pressure. Contact with serious illness and death is emotionally draining, particularly for young people. The illness and death may be visiting other people, but just observing them creates an enormous strain. It is covered by a gung-ho macabre sense of humour.

But also by alcohol.

The Hospital Hierarchy

Consultant

Senior Registrar

Registrar

Senior House Officer

House Officer (pre-registration)

Associate Specialist*

Staff Grade Specialist*

*Non-Hierarchical Jobs

A CAREER IN HOSPITAL MEDICINE

How to become a consultant

All newly-qualified doctors must do two six-month appointments in hospital, one in medicine and one in surgery. This is the pre-registration year. It is compulsory. After the satisfactory completion of that year, they receive full recognition from the General Medical Council and are allowed to practise as independent doctors outside the confines and protective umbrella of a hospital.

In terms of competence and ability newly-qualified doctors are woefully inexperienced. The only thing they have proved is that they are fit for postgraduate training.

In the United States, postgraduate training is efficiently organised. The newly-qualified doctor first spends a year as an 'intern', which is similar to the British pre-registration year. After that, the similarities end. The American doctor then applies for a residency training programme in his chosen speciality. Entrance is subject to careful screening and is not guaranteed. Residency programmes are finite in length. Once accepted on such a programme, there is an over-

whelming likelihood that the doctor will become an accredited specialist. There are residency programmes in all specialities, including family medicine or general practice. The programmes last for a varying and appropriate number of years, depending upon the speciality. At the end of the programme the doctor takes State Board exams in the speciality and if he passes them will be accepted as competent to practise.

These USA State Board exams can be described as 'exit' exams. Once passed, they enable the doctor to exit the training programme and practise as an independent specialist, or consultant. He can put up his name plate and apply to hospitals for admission rights. He can ply his trade in the medical market place and his success will depend on his competence.

Inevitably, some doctors do not get the particular residency they want, and a few unsuitable candidates are accepted. But on the whole the system works. Newly-qualified doctors choose the career they want to pursue and, subject to demonstration of reasonable likelihood of success, are admitted to a structured training programme. They emerge from the other end as properly trained and accredited specialists.

There is no such certainty in Britain. The main source of career guidance is goat-shagger's gossip.[1] Although some specialities are trying to institute formal training programmes like the residency programmes in the USA this is still the exception rather than the rule. Many newly-qualified British medical graduates just drift through a few SHO jobs whilst they see which career takes their fancy. When they do decide, they have to fight their way up an ill-defined promotion ladder from SHO to registrar to senior registrar and finally to consultant.

Their ability to succeed is dependent on their ability to climb the ladder. Unlike their American counterparts, no-one tells them where to find the ladder, and they are blindfolded before they start climbing. Many fall off on the way, and years of expensive training go to waste.

Senior registrars are a case in point. Appointments at senior registrar level are normally for a maximum of four years. After that there is no guarantee of further employment. The senior registrar who fails to find a consultancy may get a continuance but eventually will have to give way to juniors coming up behind him.

There is no sadder sight in the NHS hierarchy than the time-expired senior registrar. Despite ten or more years training, he faces the real prospect of unemployment. Once, he would have gone into general practice. He cannot do that anymore without meeting the career requirements for that speciality, and that at the very minimum will mean a trainee

---

[1] For detailed consideration of goat-shaggers see page 47

---

year and quite probably one or more years doing hospital jobs in specialities of which he has no experience, such as obstetrics or paediatrics. And *still* he may not get a job. The modern GP group practice is looking for dedicated family doctors, not rejects from other disciplines

The senior registrar who cannot get a consultancy may be forced to take one of the cul-de-sac jobs of 'staff grade specialist'. The number of foreign doctors in these posts provides strong circumstantial evidence of racial prejudice in the NHS. It's all right for these "foreign chappies" to do all the monotonous work, but they are not welcome in the golf club.

The junior ranks of the NHS are staffed by a group of people who are, in the main, committed and caring doctors. They are surrounded by thinly-veiled prejudice and discrimination. All foreign doctors suffer, and the darker their skin, the worse the prejudice. They are poorly-paid, routinely abused and have no guarantee of reaching a consultancy. For many, often foreign or female or both, the word is out on the bush-telegraph, or at the local goat-shaggers' meeting, that they are not "suitable material". No-one will ever sit down and tell them so. Everyone is charming to their faces, but behind their backs they are referred to as "hot-country doctors" or "non-reflectors". They are allowed to labour on doing all the scut work until finally they time-expire.

In summary, British medical training consists of allowing any doctor, suitable or not, to enter any form of self-organised postgraduate training. After years of hard work and poor pay, the undesirables are weeded out and shunted into non-career cul-de-sacs.

Racial and sexual prejudice are both rampant.

The Fairer Sex

Since at least half the entrants to medical schools are women it would be reasonable to expect an equal distribution of male and female consultants. Well, alright, some women will want to forgo a career to bring up their families, and we can't prevent them can we? Even though it is a waste of their training. But what is the real distribution? The table below gives the 1987 figures, and nothing's changed much since then.

Where have all the women gone? Thirty-three per cent of audiologists are female, but there are only fifteen jobs in the country. And very boring jobs they are too. Of the sensible specialities, paediatrics and haematology have the best representation. How do we explain that nearly twelve per cent of geriatricians are female but only four to five percent make it in general medicine? Why are over sixteen per cent of venereologists female but less than one per cent of general surgeons? Answers on a post card, please, to the Equal Opportunities Commission.

Royal College Rackets: *Training the Monkeys*

Postgraduate medical exams are set by the Royal Colleges. Not only is postgraduate training unstructured, but many of the Royal Colleges make no attempt to supervise the candidates entering the exams.

Males & Females in medical specialities in England & Wales, 1987

Speciality	Total	% Female
General Medicine	1,295	4.6
Cardiology	136	5.9
Gastroenterology	34	2.9
Nephrology	67	4.5
Thoracic (chest) medicine	105	8.6
Geriatric medicine	487	11.9
Audiology	15	33.3
Dermatology	237	21.1
Venereology	134	16.4
Paediatrics	660	22.4

Males & Females in medical specialities in England & Wales, 1987, contd.

General surgery	954	0.6
Orthopaedic surgery	711	0.6
Neurosurgery	98	1
Gynaecology	793	11.6
Psychiatry	1,251	18
Pathology	668	19.2
Haematology	380	21.8
Radiology	1,042	20

Figures taken from DHSS Medical Manpower and Education division (1988). Medical and dental staffing prospects in the NHS in England and Wales in 1987. Health Trends, 20, 101-9

The FRCS examination is divided into two parts. The Royal College of Surgeons allows doctors to take each part of the exam as many times as they like. But in the UK there is not just one Royal College of Surgeons. There are three; one each for England, Scotland and Ireland.

When examination time comes around, hordes of trainee surgeons 'fly the triangle' from England to Scotland and then to Ireland. Give a thousand monkeys a penknife and a copy of Gray's Anatomy, and sooner or later...

Why do the Royal Colleges allow this nonsense? Camaraderie and claret; more precisely, the price of claret.

At the time of writing, the fee for Part 1 of FRCS is one hundred and eighty-five pounds, and for Part II, three hundred and forty pounds. Doctors pay these fees out of their own pockets. The examiners meet up for the annual or biannual examination junkets to natter with old friends and colleagues, to wine and dine, and to indulge in their favourite extra-curricular activity, the humiliation of junior doctors. It's better than skeet shooting.

The Colleges receive huge revenues and can replenish their cellars.

Watering down the Beer

If examination revenue is to be maximised, the exam must be taken by as many candidates as possible. It should therefore be taken early in the career and have a high failure rate. Exams taken early in careers cannot be a mark of experience.

Many long-standing and once-proud qualifications have been thoroughly degraded over the years and now serve as no more than entrance exams to higher professional training.

Fellowship of the Royal College of Surgeons is an excellent example. Once a doctor can put FRCS after his name he drops his courtesy title of 'Doctor' and becomes 'Mister'. The layman thinks this means he is a competent and qualified surgeon.

Not true.

He may not be able to remove an appendix. Many London hospitals have tiny catchment areas and so attract little emergency out-of-hours surgery. When the occasional patient with abdominal pain does arrive, the junior surgeons, all with FRCS, are queuing to open him up.

MRCP (Membership of the Royal College of Physicians) is even more meaningless. Not only is it an entrance exam for higher professional training in general medicine, but other specialities use it as their entrance exam. It is difficult to get into radiology without MRCP or FRCS, and as MRCP is the easier exam, that is the usual one taken.

If the prospective patient is to gauge how competent and experienced a doctor is likely to be, he must understand the real significance of medical qualifications. In particular, are they entrance or exit exams?

The tables on the following pages will help you strain the alphabet soup and find the competent doctors.

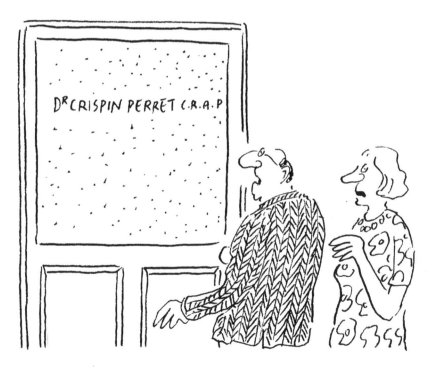

"Look on the bright side Cynth– at least he's got *some* letters after his name."

Medical qualifications – a consumer's guide

Qualification	Translation	Type	Experience needed	Comments
THE BASIC QUALIFICATIONS				
MB Bs MB ChB MB BChir	Bachelor of medicine and surgery – a university degree	Entrance exam; the first hurdle	None whatsoever	Circumstantial evidence of fitness to start medical training
MRCS LRCP	Member of the Royal College of Surgeons and Licentiate of the Royal College of Physicians	Entrance exam set by the Royal Colleges A revenue generator	Even less than for the university degree except in surgery where some knowledge of anatomy is required	Ditto above. Doctors who put these letters after their name as well as university degrees are ostentatious wallies
LMSSA*	The Society of Apothecaries	Entrance exam	None	Holders of this qualification believe they have the ancient right to ask a City of London police officer to shelter them whilst they pee over London Bridge

*From January 1994 the Society of Apothecaries and the Conjoint Board will be merging to set a unified final exam, and will be known as the United Examination Board. As both wish to retain their examination identity, and an Act of Parliament is needed to change medical qualifications, the successful candidates of the unified exam will be entitled to put 'LMSSA Lond LRCP Lond LRCS Eng' after their name. What a lot of letters.

Qualification	Translation	Type	Experience needed	Comments

POSTGRADUATE QUALIFICATIONS

Qualification	Translation	Type	Experience needed	Comments
MRCP	Membership of the Royal College of Physicians	Entrance	Not much these days	Needs to get its act together; so devalued now that other specialities use it as an entrance exam to their training courses
FRCP	Fellowship of the Royal College of Physicians	Not an exam at all – awarded by the College for being a good chap	Serial goat-shagging	Not many women get it, so to speak
FRCS	Fellowship of the Royal College of Surgeons	Entrance	Lancing boils and anal stretches	A sadly devalued exam. Allows progression to higher surgical training.
MRCOG/ FRCOG (automatic progression to Fellowship)	Membership or Fellowship of the Royal College of Obstetricians and Gynaecologists	Mid-way between entrance and exit	Defined jobs & experience needed – ability to do a hysterectomy and deliver a baby at the very least	Gynaecologists call themselves Mister as they like to pretend they are real surgeons

Qualification	Translation	Type	Experience needed	Comments
FFARCS	Fellow of the Faculty of Anaesthetics of the Royal College of Surgeons (not grown up enough to have their own college)	Mid-way between entrance and exit. Shows ability to put a patient to sleep with a chance that he may wake up after the operation	Defined job-experience needed	"The gas man cometh." Everyone ridicules anaesthetists who are regarded as failed surgeons. Unfair. Many of them are failed physicians.
FRCR	Fellow of the Royal College of Radiologists	Exit exam	Wide and defined specialist training needed	The RCR has got its act together. The nearest to US-style residency training in NHS
FRCPath	Fellow of the Royal College of Pathologists	Exit exam	Lots. Almost guarantees a consultancy and rightly so	Who wants to do a job like this though?
MRCGP	Membership of the Royal College of General Practitioners	Beyond classification; no-one knows what it measures	Who knows?	So many GPs hold the qualification in contempt that it may actually hinder a career
M(F)RCPSCHY	Membership or Fellowship of the Royal College of Psychiatrists	Mid-way between entrance and exit exam	Evidence of ability to communi-cate with other psychiatrists	Branded for life – holders would have difficulty changing to another speciality

Qualification	Translation	Type	Experience needed	Comments
ACADEMIC POSTGRADUATE TRAINING				
MD (DM from Oxbridge)	Doctor of Medicine	A bit of class, that's all	Two years churning out meaningless research papers, few of which are published and even fewer read	Increasingly a requirement for a consultant post. The academic qualification that provides the title 'Doctor'.
MS	Master of Surgery	A bit of class, that's all	Same as an MD but designed for surgeons	Increasingly required for a consultant post
PhD (DPhil from Oxbridge)	Doctor of Philosophy	Lots of class	Three years research – much more difficult than MDs which come off a production line	Stuffy academics who have no interest in patients

```
┌─────────────────────────────┐
│                             │
│   DIPLOMAS                  │
│                             │
└─────────────────────────────┘
```

As well as all the qualifications in the tables, patients should be aware of the wide variety of medical *diplomas*. They look plausible. The main ones are:

> • DRCOG - The Diploma of the Royal College of Obstetricians and Gynaecologists

The majority of holders are GPs. To take the exam they must have had experience of both subjects and the only sensible way to acquire such experience is to have held a substantive appointment in a hospital.

Holders of this qualification will usually automatically qualify to be 'on the obstetric list' of their FHSA and will get higher payments for providing ante-natal care to their patients.

> • DCH - Diploma of Child Health

Again designed for GPs. A difficult examination requiring considerable academic knowledge. Now oriented more towards community paediatrics.

> • FPCert - Certificate of Family Planning

Definite evidence of theoretical and practical training in family planning. But watch out. No compulsion to update the certificate. Not much use if taken twenty years ago. Could be dangerous.

Quality not Quantity

The ability of a doctor may be reflected in his qualifications but his pomposity is inversely proportional to his desire to display them. Consider:

Dr John Smith MD FRCP

Consultant Physician

St Elsewhere's Hospital

---

and

Dr Peter Jones

MB ChB MRCS LRCP LMSSA MRCGP DRCOG DCH

Medical Aromatherapist and Allergist

The Allergy & Aromatherapy Centre

Wimpole Street

Who is the more qualified? Dr Smith only has six letters after his name, but they have class. Yes, to get an FRCP he may be a goat-shagger, but he also has an MD and is a consultant physician in an NHS hospital, albeit St Elsewheres.

It will have taken him a minimum of ten years postgraduate training to get these important six letters. He may well have an MRCS LRCP and a diploma or two but he is not vulgar enough to display them.

Dr Jones, however, displays the lot. The first three qualifications are duplications and the final four - thirteen letters in all - could be acquired with three years' experience at very junior level.

Dr Smith may be an incompetent twerp and Dr Jones a genius. Or vice versa. But where would you take your sick grandmother?

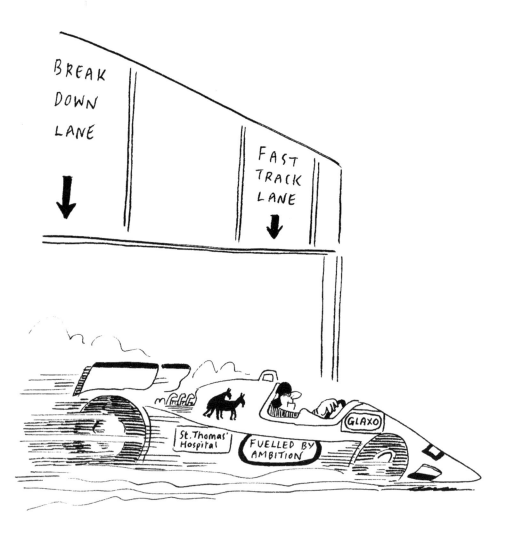

CLIMBING
THE GREASY POLE

"There are only two sorts of doctors: those who practise with their brains, and those who practise with their tongues."

SIR WILLIAM OSLER (1849-1919)

Of Golf and Goat-Shagging

Doctors can be divided into two groups. Those who are involved in goat-shagging, and those who are not.

In a perfect world, career preferment would depend entirely upon ability. There is no profession in which this is true, but there is none worse than medicine for considering factors which the average person would regard as irrelevant.

Sex, class and racial origin remain crucial factors. Academic ability is a secondary consideration. Provided a doctor is charming with the patient and subservient to his bosses, and provided that he passes the necessary postgraduate exams within an ill-defined but 'reasonable' timescale, it is assumed that he is a capable doctor.

What matters is his skill at brown-nosing. His clubability. One of the best ways to develop these talents is by joining the goat-shaggers.

To become a goat-shagger, a doctor has to join the Masons. This is not to suggest that Masons are in any way involved in the unlawful carnal knowledge of goats; or the lawful carnal knowledge of goats for that matter, if such an activity exists. No-one knows what the Masons get up to, and if people want to meet behind closed doors to perform ancient secret rituals, that is a matter for them.

Masonry is strong and influential in medicine. Some of the London teaching hospitals have their own Lodges, which meet at the medical school, and list many of the consultants amongst their members. The junior doctor invited to join declines at the peril of his career. The junior doctor *not* invited to join may not have a career; or not one beyond rheumatology or geriatrics.

Doctors who have not been invited to join a Lodge refer to their Masonic colleagues as goat-shaggers. This is an unpleasant and wholly inaccurate description of the activities of Masons. Those who use it are merely showing frustration at their inability to rise to the top of their profession. They are inadequates who should not have gone into medicine in the first place.

Women are not allowed to be goat-shaggers.

An alternative course to preferment is golf. And in this context course is the correct word. When you are told that your doctor has had to cancel your appointment because he is on a course, it is not his medical handicap that he is improving. The wise doctor is both a golfer and a goat-shagger.

Women are now allowed to join most of the leading golf clubs although they do not play from the same tees or in the same groups as the men. And golf clubs have taken a lead in stamping out racial prejudice. There are many more Asian and African golfers than there are goat-shaggers.

The Medical Hierarchy:
which way does the shit flow?

The clinical medical student soon learns that he is at the bottom of the pile. His desire to learn is stimulated by the need to avoid ritual public humiliation and tempered only by the social requirement of not appearing to know too much.

As he progresses up the hierarchy, the need never to be caught becomes an obsession. Doctors are deeply insecure. Most have an irrational but entrenched belief that all their colleagues are more knowledgeable than they are. And so, catching out colleagues is reassuring. Each time a doctor can do it, he feels that he is not alone in having gaps in his knowledge. But what starts at the beginning of the career as a source of reassurance, with time becomes a source of pleasure. Put a group of doctors together and within minutes the conversation turns to absent friends and their cock-ups. This is human nature. All professionals to it to some extent. But to the medical profession it is an essential part of working life.

Catching out junior doctors or medical students is too easy to provide reassurance, but it is still good sport and everyone does it as they rise through the hierarchy.

The consistent humiliation to which clinical medical students are subjected affects them for life. Ignatious Loyola wanted seven years to mould a child. The medical profession does it in three.

It is like child abuse. The abused become abusers. Georgina will be savaged particularly by the consultant surgeons. She will leave ward rounds in tears. She will spend long hours in the library desperately trying to ensure she is never caught out. And as time goes by she will be caught out less and less and will earn the grudging respect of the consultants. But the damage has already been done. When she becomes a consultant she will have an encyclopaedic

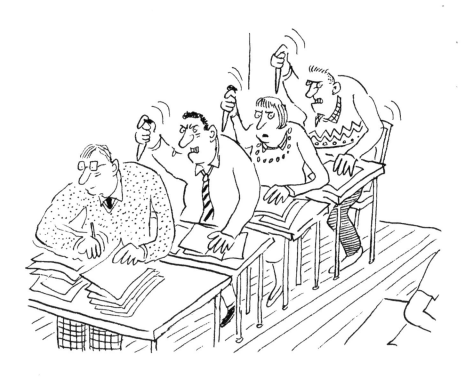

knowledge of medicine. She will have forgotten that there was a time when she did not know very much and will herself take poisonous pleasure in the humiliation of students. She will specialise in taking apart the Ruperts.

Rupert hates the humiliation but his public school veneer enables him to take it on the chin with apparent good humour. Beneath his veneer he is, like many public school boys, a sexist and immature, emotional cripple. But at medical school he is "one of the boys". He plays for the 1st XV. He has medical machismo. He hates Georgina because she is cleverer than he, and so he makes snide

remarks about the size of her breasts, often not quite out of earshot. If he becomes a consultant surgeon, he will specialise in taking apart the Georginas. And so it goes on.

Doctors not only take delight in criticising juniors; they also criticise other doctors who are theoretically at an equal level but are perceived as being inferior because they are in a different speciality. All doctors believe that their own career choice has led them to the most important and valuable position in medicine and they view other doctors from this self-appointed pinnacle.

The general physicians criticise

the general surgeons for being mindless cobblers and the general surgeons criticise the general physicians for being ineffectual; but over a glass of claret, both agree that their two specialities are at the top of the tree. In the teaching hospitals, the grand ward rounds done by these people remain in the realms of theatrical performance. It is the grandiose but pathetic behaviour of a species facing extinction: medicine and surgery have become too specialised for the generalist.

As far as the general physicians are concerned, cardiologists, nephrologists, gastroenterologists and neurologists are all respected and have considerable machismo. They are still regarded as real doctors, and it is honourable to have ambitions in these fields. As far as the general surgeons are concerned, acceptable sub-specialties are cardio-thoracic and urological surgery. Orthopaedics scrapes in if there is a history of success on the rugby field to explain the neanderthal appearance of most orthopods.

And then there are the less prestigious sub-sepcialiities: Physicians not perceived to be aiming for the top go into diabetology, endocrinology, and chest medicine; surgeons go into ENT and ophthalmology. They may still be allowed to eat at top table with their superior colleagues if they pay meticulous attention to goat-shagging. But for the rest – well, they are certainly not acknowledged as equals whatever the Hippocratic Oath might say.They may not even be allowed to join in the goat-shagging.

The pecking order after the physicians and surgeons goes:

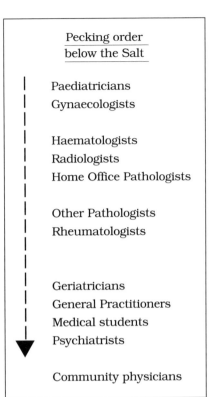

Pecking order below the Salt

| Paediatricians
| Gynaecologists
|
| Haematologists
| Radiologists
| Home Office Pathologists
|
| Other Pathologists
| Rheumatologists
|
| Geriatricians
| General Practitioners
| Medical students
| Psychiatrists

Community physicians

This ranking is deeply engrained in the medical psyche, but the casual observer might be unaware of it. Just as Her Majesty the Queen from time to time talks to one of her footmen, so, for example, the general surgeon will talk to the radiologist.

Because he wants something. The result of the most recent barium enema on one of the private patients, perhaps. Of course the general surgeon knows he could do a barium enema himself if he wanted, but he doesn't want; pouring chalky slop up patients' bottoms is not his idea of being a doctor.

The most extraordinary relationship is that between consultants and

GPs. Junior hospital doctors treat GPs with contempt. They place them somewhere on the evolutionary scale between estate agents and male hairdressers. But not consultants. To them, GPs are "colleagues". They are treated as equals and welcomed, indeed encouraged, to be active goatshaggers. GPs respond by talking about their "consultantcolleagues"[1]

What is going on? Have hospital doctors finally recognised the value of vocational training for general practice and are they now accepting that GPs are true specialists in their own right?

No. Not at all.

Like the juniors, consultants think GPs are contemptible; worse even than rheumatologists and geriatricians. In fact, consultants rank GPs below medical students, because medical students are at least able to learn.

Consultants are polite to GPs because, for the majority of them, the success or failure of their private practice is entirely in the hands of GPs.

More recently, a second factor has come into play: fundholding GPs from large practices have purchasing power. Purchasing power which can make the difference between profit and loss to a hospital. Not only do consultants have to treat these GPs with respect, but an entirely new phenomenon has arisen. The hospital administrators have to treat them with respect as well.

---

[1] 'Consultantcolleague' is a concept not a phrase. During their vocational training GPs are taught to say it as one word.

The Yellow Brick Road - a trip down Harley Street

'A physician who heals for nothing is worth nothing.'

THE TALMUD

Private practice is the life blood of the NHS consultant. The BMA fought the introduction of the NHS in 1948 tooth and nail. It might not have started at all had the Labour Government not conceded the right for doctors appointed to NHS consultancies to have private patients as well.

A doctor does not have to be either in the NHS or have risen to the rank of consultant to have private patients. There is nothing to stop junior hospital doctors seeing patients privately; or nothing in the law, at least. A few senior registrars do have the odd private patient. All juniors are of course attuned to looking after the bosses' private patients both when he is on holiday or on a 'course'.

NHS consultants can choose to be full-time or what is called 'maximum part time'. It works like this. The medical week is divided into ten sessions. A notional eleventh session is added to cover administrative work, work done over lunch hours and thinking about work when in the shower. Once a consultant's private earnings are more than ten per cent of his NHS salary, it is assumed that his private practice must be interfering with his NHS work, and he is obliged to go 'maximum part time'. His NHS salary is reduced by one eleventh. A one-eleventh reduction taken from fifty thousand pounds is not a problem for the cardiac surgeon with private fees of over two hundred and fifty thousand pounds a year. To a haematologist who earns only five thousand pounds a year privately, the cut is very serious.

So, the consultant with the large private practice has his NHS salary reduced by one eleventh. A fair deal for the taxpayer? Hardly. If his juniors to do all his NHS work whilst he is on Harley Street, his salary should be reduced by ten elevenths, or he should not be paid at all.

The super-rich consultants are at least consistent. They do not just abuse the NHS. They abuse private patients as well. They build up a team of "assistants" who are junior doctors doing research; their salaries are paid by medical schools or by the NHS. "Research" in this case means seeing the consultant's private patients. Sometimes, the consultant is so rich that he can afford to pay a junior doctor's salary himself, to "help" with the private work.

Two classes of private patients emerge. The upper class are seen by the consultant himself; the lower class are seen by one of his private assistants.

The UPPER CLASS

• **The rich and famous**. They flatter the consultant's ego and also help to spread his reputation in the right circles.

• **Foreigners**. They pay whatever the consultant demands, rather than just the standard scales agreed with the private health insurance companies. The Harley Street rip-off of Middle East patients reached such a level in the nineteen eighties that even the oil-rich Arabs started to notice the size of the bills. Many decided to take their business to Germany where there are more doctors and lower charges.

• **GPs and their immediate family**, for obvious reasons. No charge is made but a case of claret is expected.

The LOWER CLASS

• **All the rest**. They have health insurance and the bills they pay are set by national agreements with the private health insurance companies. They cannot be milked.

The lower-class private patient is being ripped off. He has paid through the nose to buy health insurance so that he is not treated by one of those junior doctors who is still learning and he ends up being treated by one of those junior doctors who is still learning. But because it is a posh private clinic with leather armchairs, Country Life and soft lavatory paper, and because the junior doctor is wearing a clean white coat, or, more likely still, no white coat at all, the patient is fooled. If he found out what is going on he would be angry. He rarely does.

The greatest irony of all is that there is a double bluff here. Although he would never believe it, the lower-class private patient may be getting *better* treatment than the upper-class patient. It is often safer to see the junior doctor who is more thorough, more conscientious, more interested in the subject and, most important of all, has more up-to-date experience than the consultant.

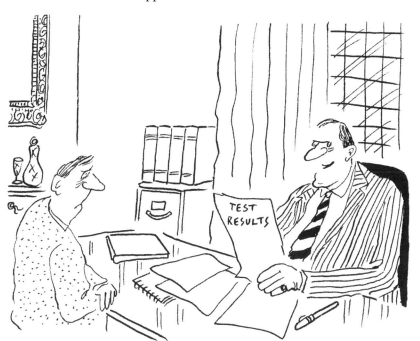

"The *good* news? Oh yes. You know that little blonde receptionist you saw on your way in. Well last night I finally screwed her!"

Passing the Golden Baton

When a new consultant is appointed he may be lucky enough to be handed the private list of his predecessor. More often, one of two things happens:

1. His predecessor will have retired only from the NHS and will continue to milk his private practice for as long as he gets referrals. He may even write to all the GPs in the area to say that he is still available to see private patients. This does not work for long. GPs have a deep-seated prejudice against private referrals to consultants who do not also see NHS patients.

2. Other consultants in the same speciality will steal the private patients before he has a chance to meet them.

So the new consultant may start with only a few scraps of private practice. The first thing he will do is send his card to all the GPs in the area:

Mr David J. Hopefull MS FRCS

Consultant ENT Surgeon

presents his compliments and wishes to advise you that he is available to see private patients at

The Clinic
3, The Yellow Brick Road
LONDON W1

Efficient GPs file this card under 'ENT surgeons: private'. The concept of an efficient GP is an oxymoron and most of these cards end up in the bin.

Even so, no tears should be shed on Mr Hopeful's account. He will have no problem at all finding patients as there is a desperate shortage of NHS ENT surgeons. Parents will always find the money to pay for a private operation on their children rather than wait eighteen months on the NHS. Within a couple of years, Dr Hopeful will quadruple his NHS salary, and ultimately the rewards will be even higher.

The same is true of any field involving operations that are in demand. The financially ambitious doctor chooses a speciality that has lots of little operations, or even lots of *one little* operation like the ophthalmologist and cataract extractions. Ideally, they should be operations for non-life threatening conditions, and be elective. Middle-class patients like having elective procedures.[1] The common folk who do not have private insurance find the waiting lists on the NHS so long that the condition either gets better by itself or they learn to live with it and cannot be bothered to have the operation.

The biggest earner of all is the cardiac surgeon. His operations last three to four hours or more, but he charges three thousand pounds a go.

---

[1] An elective procedure is one which patients choose to undergo to remedy a troublesome but non-life-threatening condition: stripping varicose veins; straightening crooked noses; removing benign but ugly moles, and so on.

He can do three CABGs[2] a week comfortably. If he is a fat cat, he may do many more. Of course, he does not actually *do* the operations. The juniors crack the chest open and then call him on his mobile; he arrives in the operating theatre, replaces the blocked arteries, and leaves twenty minutes later. The "boys" are left to tidy up the patient (i.e. put him back together again) and at the end of the month the consultant will slip them fifty quid. Net profit for less than an hour's work; two thousand nine hundred pounds. No wonder they do not care about merit awards.

Can private GPs give value for money?

NHS GPs are allowed to have private patients but few can survive on private practice alone. There are restrictions on the private services a GP may offer. Those restrictions rebound more on the patient than the doctor, making the perceived status of having a private GP an expensive luxury.

A GP is not allowed to offer any private service to an NHS patient. The private patient must first be removed from the NHS list. Once removed, the private patient cannot receive NHS prescriptions and will have to pay the full market price of all his medication.

In return for this sacrifice, the private patient is looking for instant availability of his own doctor and preferably his home phone number. Few get it. Out-of-hours, they have to phone the deputising service, or the co-operative, like everyone else.

During the day, the conscientious GP is already seeing patients with urgent problems as quickly as he can. What more can he do for the private patient? How, in all conscience, can he offer the private patient a service he does not provide for the NHS patient?

Under current regulations, the NHS GP with private patients is either offering an inferior service to his NHS patients, and may be in breach of his terms and conditions of service for so doing, or he is ripping off his private patients by charging them for services he provides to others for free.

---

[2] 'Coronary artery bypass grafts'

HOW MUCH
DO DOCTORS EARN?

Hush Money

The Hippocratic Oath states the traditional obligations imposed upon and the proper conduct required from those intending to be physicians.

It does not mention private practice; nor private health insurance; nor even allude to the concept of a fair salary. Splendid stuff indeed. Now we know why doctors' sons get into medical school so easily. Few people realise that doctors do not take the Hippocratic Oath. They never have.

The Hippocratic Oath

'I swear by Apollo the physician, by Aesculapius, Hygeia, and Panacea, and I take to witness all the gods, all the goddesses, to keep according to my ability and my judgement the following Oath:

To consider dear to me as my parents him who taught me this art; to live in common with him and if necessary to share my goods with him; to look upon his children as my own brothers, to teach them this art if they so desire without fee or written promise; to impart to my sons and the sons of the master who taught me and the disciples who have enrolled themselves and have agreed to the rules of the progression, but to these alone, the precepts and the instruction. I will prescribe regimen for the good of my patients according to my ability and my judgement and never do harm to anyone. To please no one will I prescribe a deadly drug, nor give advice which may cause his death. Nor will I give a woman a pessary to procure abortion. But I will preserve the purity of my life and my art. I will not cut for stone, even for patients in whom the disease is manifest: I will leave this operation to be performed by practitioners (specialists in this art). In every house where I come I will enter only for the good of my patients, keeping myself far from all intentional ill-doing and all seduction, and especially from the pleasures of love with women or with men be they free or slaves. All that may come to my knowledge in the exercise of my profession or outside of my profession or in daily commerce with men, which ought not to be spread abroad, I will keep secret and will never reveal. If I keep this oath faithfully, may I enjoy my life and practise my art, respected by all men and in all times; but if I swerve from it or violate it, may the reverse be my lot.'

The whole concept of paying doctors is seen - by doctors at any rate - as really rather vulgar. By vulgar, they mean it is better not talked about. Provided the money is right.

So let's talk about it now.

In Britain, the remuneration of all doctors comes from two sources. From the NHS and/or from private practice. It is difficult to work entirely in the private sector without holding a contemporaneous NHS appointment. Some manage it. Of those who do, many are reputable. Some are not. A patient paying to see such a doctor should scrutinise his qualifications and experience very carefully.

Hospital doctors and GPs are paid in entirely different ways. Here's how it works:

GPs

When the NHS started in 1948 it would have been logical to have had both hospital doctors and GPs on a salary. This was strongly opposed by the BMA who wished to protect the self-employed independent contractor status of all doctors. A dual compromise was reached. Consultants were to be allowed to continue in private practice as well holding a health service appointment; GPs would remain self-employed, although bound by Terms and Conditions of Service enforced by local Family Practitioner Committees (now called Family Health Service Authorities - FHSAs).

This independent contractor status of the self-employed GP has made the pay system labyrinthinely complicated.

First of all, the GP is paid a Basic Practice Allowance (BPA), provided he is full-time and provided he has a certain number of patients. In this context 'full-time' means working a minimum of twenty-six hours a week. On top of the BPA, he receives a capitation fee for each patient which rises with the age of the patient. Then there are allowances for seniority (time-serving) and for maintaining postgraduate education. Target payments will be made if a certain proportion of the GP's list have had smears and appropriate immunisations and there are financial incentives for defined health-promotion work.

In addition, the GP may earn money from what are called 'items-of-service' which are a form of piece work. For example, each girl he puts on the pill will earn him £13.25 a year and each patient for whom he provides complete maternity care a maximum of £165.05. (see table overleaf)

It might be thought possible for the astute GP to earn unlimited sums of money by working harder and harder. Not so. For the government maintains a pool system. At the beginning of each financial year, it decides what a GP's average net remuneration should be. For 1994 this is £40,610. It then sets aside an amount of money sufficient to pay that figure on a national basis, and juggles all the respective payments so that the average GP can achieve it. Of course, some earn more and some earn less. But if the profession as a whole works harder that expected and earns a total sum which on a national basis exceeds the amount put in the pool that amount of money will be paid but then clawed back the following year. GPs are thus in the unique position of being financially penalised for hard work.

GPs may also have private patients. Some do. Most do not. All of them receive private fees for insurance reports and private medicals.

So what does the average GP really earn? When all sources of income are taken into account, more than the government's intended net remuneration, that's for sure. The range of pay is enormous, probably varying from as low as twenty thousand pounds for the struggling, often foreign, inner-city single-handed doctor with a very small list to as high as a hundred thousand pounds for the slick, Home Counties, business-oriented doctor who is running three

nursing homes. The majority of GPs at present earn fifty thousand pounds per year, plus or minus twenty per cent.

Thus, if we leave aside consultants' merit awards,[1] and private practice, many GPs are earning more than consultants in hospital practice. And bear in mind that GPs reach their maximum earning potential much quicker than consultants. It takes four years postgraduate training to become a GP principal. It may take fourteen years to become a consultant.

The ultimate financial rewards of hospital medicine are immense if a lucrative speciality is chosen, but over a lifetime's earnings, the GP's total income compares well with that of the average hospital consultant.

[1] GPs are not eligible for Merit Awards. Only consultants are. See page 63.

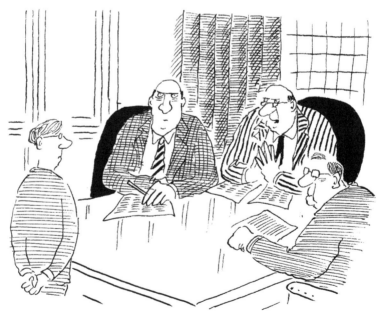

"We practise medicine to make money Watkins. If you can think of a better reason, let's hear it."

Summary of GP Remuneration

Basic Practice Allowance (For a minimum of 1,200 patients)	£6,624
Annual Capitation Fees (i.e. for each patient) Under 65 65-74 75 plus	 £14.30 £18.85 £36.45
Seniority Payments 7 years 14 years 5 years	 £415.00 £2,165.00 £4,665.00
Target Payments Child immunisations Cervical Smears Health Promotion	 £1,860.0 £2,355.00 £2,105.00
Items of Service (piece rate, per patient per year) Contraception IUCD (Coil) fitting Complete ante-natal care Night visit (by self) Night visit (by deputy)	 £13.25 £44.35 £165.05 £46.65 £15.55

Hospital Doctors

As one would expect, pay within the hospital service depends upon seniority. At the bottom of the pile is the newly-qualified doctor who has to do two six-month appointments in recognised hospitals, one in medicine and one in surgery. He is the House Officer, or gopher.

After that year he attains full registration and rises up the ladder to Senior House Officer, Registrar, Senior Registrar and finally Consultant.

Depending upon the speciality he chooses, he may spent two, three or even four years at each level, not attaining a consultancy until he has been qualified for anything between ten and twenty years. The salary scale for each of these appointments is summarised in the table below. The

Hospital Doctor Pay Guide for Career Posts (from April 1994)

House Officer*	£13,950
Senior House Officer	£16,960
Year 2	£18,100
Year 3	£19,240
Year 4	£20,380
Year 5	£21,520
Registrar	£19,223
Year 2	£20,200
Year 3	£21,175
Year 4	£22,150
Year 5	£23,325
Senior Registrar	£22,150
Year 2	£23,325
Year 3	£24,500
Year 4	£25,675
Year 5	£26,850
Year 6	£28,025
Consultant	£39,625
Year 2	£42,510
Year 3	£45,395
Year 4	£48,280
Year 5	£51,165

*House Officers are only provisionally registered as doctors. They can only work within hospitals, notionally under supervision. On successful completion of the first year they will get full registration and will automatically get SHO status.

starting salary at each level is given together with the annual increments.

Thus, the most junior doctor, the house officer, earns a basic £13,590 and the most senior, a consultant with five years or more experience at that level, earns £51,165.

A new post has recently been created within the hospital service – that of 'Associate Specialist'.

This is one of the 'non-career' posts designed for doctors who want to work in hospital medicine, but who don't want to become consultants. Allegedly. In fact, just as nobody becomes an MP without ambitions to achieve office, nobody goes into hospital medicine without ambitions to become a consultant.

Non-career posts in hospital medicine

Associate Specialist
£23,500 - £40,880

Staff grade practitioner
£21,200 - £31,580

The truth is that these posts have been created for doctors who are not able to become consultants either because they are not capable, or because, and this is the more common situation, the system has discriminated against them.

This means that associate specialists are frustrated. Most of them are foreign. Or female. Or both. They are treated like drones. They get all the jobs that no-one else wants to do. For example, a gynaecology associate specialist is likely to be doing all the abortions in the hospital.

Other Income for Hospital Doctors

There are three other sources of income for the hospital practitioner. Overtime, Merit Awards (consultants only) and Private Practice. The first two are dealt with in this chapter, and private practice in Chapter Seven.

OVERTIME

Overtime payments can be earned by junior hospital doctors (i.e. house officer to senior registrar level) but not by consultants or associate specialists. Although the rates are miserly, and would certainly not be tolerated by any trades union, the hours worked by the juniors are so long that the total amount earned can be considerable.

A senior registrar at the top of his grade will earn £28,025 basic salary but may get another £15,000 in overtime payments. When he gets a consultancy, his starting salary will rise to £39,625 but he won't be able to earn anuthing on overtime. In other words, promotion to the top job involves a substantial pay cut. No wonder morale in the NHS is low.

Overtime is classified into Additional Duty Hours (ADHs). From February 1992 additional duty hours contracted beyond the basic 40 per week are paid at the following percentages of basic salary:

Full shift – 100% of basic pay

Partial shift – 70% of basic pay

On-call rota – 50% of basic pay

Thus, even when working on Christmas Day, the junior hospital doctor will never get an overtime rate higher than his basic salary rate.

But it gets worse. The employers - i.e. the hospitals, many of which are now independent trusts and obliged to make a profit - rarely accept that a doctor has to do extra 'full-shift' work outside the normal forty-hour week. Most additional work is classified as 'on-call rota' and paid at 50% overtime rate. For the dermatology senior registrar who does his on-call from home and is only likely to be called into the hospital for a dermatological emergency this is a very good deal indeed. Dermatological emergencies occur less frequently than leap years.

In less esoteric specialities such as medicine, surgery or obstetrics, being on-call means being in the hospital working non-stop. For these unfortunates, particularly the house officer, on-call is often busier than the routine working week, and particularly so on Bank Holidays when the rest of the hospital is closed, and they have to cover for everyone else.

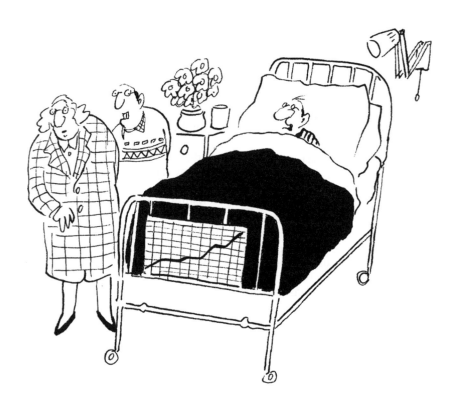

"Oh that's nothing to do with me. It's my consultant's salary."

MERIT AWARDS

The merit award system was set up with the best of intentions but has become the greatest financial scandal in the NHS.

The rationale is fine: consultants whose clinical work is of particular merit, or those who have shouldered administrative tasks beyond the boundaries of their contractual responsibilities, should receive additional remuneration. So far so good. Few would quarrel with that. The maximum NHS salary a senior consultant in London can earn is £51,165. A lot of money, perhaps. But a senior partner in a London firm of accountants or solicitors earns £200,000 or more as does a senior doctor in the USA or Canada. Why should the successful British doctor, at the top of his profession, be so relatively poorly rewarded?

The merit award system was meant to be the solution. By all means let us reward industry. Let us stop the brain drain to America. Let us, indeed, reward merit.

Unfortunately, merit is not the criterion used for selecting the recipients of awards. It is more a question of where you work and who you know. Above all else, time-serving counts.

The system is shrouded in secrecy. Few members of the public have heard of it, and it is not possible to find out who has and who has not received a merit award.

The awards are made by local committees of doctors and administrators sitting in secret. The goatshaggers are influential. The committee does not have to explain its decisions and cannot be called to account. Lists of recipients are not published.

Once a merit award has been given it is unlikely to be taken away. It is added to the salary every year for life and, most importantly, is taken into account when calculating pensions.

There are 4 levels of merit awards:

A+ awards	£48,605
A awards	£35,815
B awards	£20,465
C awards	£10,235

Remember, these are **annual** payments to consultants on top of their NHS salaries. In November 1993 it was reported that nearly seven thousand consultants in the UK held merit awards. The cost to the country is a staggering eighty million pounds. Although names of holders are unavailable, the distribution of each level of award is published.

Distribution of Merit Awards (1993)

A+ awards	232
A awards	802
B awards	1789
C awards	4102

'A+' holders are likely to be teaching hospital professors and Deans of medical schools. This is sometimes

64

explained by the fact that they have
limited opportunities for private practice, and are obliged to pass what
private fees they do earn on to their
departments. It is not a very convinc-
ing argument, for three reasons.

In the first place, some professors only accept their academic appointments on the understanding that
they *can* keep their private earnings.

In the second place, when they
do pass on private income to their
departments, it goes into what is
known in the trade as the "slush
fund". Some of it is undoubtedly spent
on research. But was that Professor
Jones I saw on the Orient Express?
And wasn't that Professor Smith and
his family skiing in Meribel? Of course
they are both giving lunchtime lectures, but who is paying for the holiday? Benefits in kind are not as good
as income paid into a personal bank
account, but at least there is none of
that nasty income tax.

The third reason why the explanation lacks conviction goes to the
very root of merit awards. They were
supposed to reward *merit*, not compensate for lack of private earnings.
The fact that a professor is not making as much privately as he could is
not a reason to bless him with huge
public hand-outs.

'A' merit awards go to other teaching hospital consultants. 'B's and 'C's
will be more scattered.

Thus, a consultant at the top of
his pay scale with, say, a 'B' merit
award will be earning £71,630 from
the NHS before he has started his
private practice. (The possibilities of
private practice are dealt with in Chapter Seven.)

The Bottom Line

British doctors are not poor. They
have many non-monetary compen-
sations. They have status in the community, though less than in years
gone by. They are recession-proof.
They are virtually unsackable unless
they start sleeping with their patients.
On the other hand, they are badly
paid compared to their colleagues in
America or to city lawyers and accountants in the UK.

And so, to the aspiring doctor; if
money is your sole interest, don't do
medicine. Or do it in the USA. Otherwise, be a lawyer or an accountant.

If you must go into medicine and
want to stay in the UK, and are still
interested in a high income, either
make sure you have the skill, luck
and patience to become a consultant
in a lucrative speciality such as
gynaecology; or become a GP as soon
as possible in a high-earning practice
which owns and runs nursing homes.

HOW HARD DO DOCTORS WORK?

Consultants

A hospital consultant is contracted to work a forty-hour week and also to provide whatever out-of-hours cover is necessary and appropriate in his speciality. That is all. He does not clock on or off and, in the absence of complaints, no-one checks on what he does.

The cynical teaching hospital consultant with a large compliment of junior staff may spend the whole of the normal working week on Harley Street seeing private patients. He is still paid ten-elevenths of his NHS salary. He will rarely be called out at night because he has a highly experienced registrar or senior registrar who can cope just as well if not better with emergencies. What is more, the juniors soon learn that the boss does not like to be called and that he will treat any such call as a sign of incompetence.

In 1979 the author was a house officer for a leading London consultant surgeon. During the author's three-month appointment, the consultant did not attend *a single* NHS ward round nor *a single* NHS operating list. The junior staff were left to cope on their own. The author had only one contact with the consultant when he was asked to leave the NHS operating list where he was assisting the registrar and go immediately to the private block to assist at a private operation.

This consultant was earning a minimum £51,165 from the NHS on today's terms. He probably had a merit award. He also had one of the largest private practices in the country and was unlikely to be earning less than £250,000 in private fees.

Consultants such as this are defrauding the NHS of both their salary and their merit award.

At the other extreme, the conscientious consultant in the provinces who has no experienced junior staff may be in the hospital three or four nights a week and most weekends. He will not have anything like as large a private practice as his London colleague and is unlikely to have a merit award unless he is about to retire. If he does have one, it will only be a 'C'.

In 1993, the entire consultant staff in the X-Ray department of a famous London teaching hospital were admonished by the Royal College of Radiologists. Their absenteeism from their NHS commitments was so great that not only were the junior doctors doing all the NHS work, they were not even receiving any postgraduate education or supervision.

The majority of consultants are conscientious and do not abuse their position. However large their private practice, they still devote a full forty hours a week, often more, to their NHS commitments. And remember, although the change in status to maximum part-time reduces their pay by one-eleventh, it does not correspondingly reduce their NHS commitment. The gross abusers are few in number but, as is so often the case, they attract a disproportionate amount of comment. It remains to be seen whether some of the stricter regulations introduced by the Trust hospitals, such as clinical directorates and job plans, will bring these erring few to order.

GPs

The most onerous aspect of being a GP is that there is a contractual responsibility to provide medical care for patients twenty-four hours a day, three hundred and sixty-five days a year.

This responsibility may be shared with partners, or delegated to another doctor or deputy, but the GP himself will always retain overall responsibility for his list of patients.

Having said that, the GP who is full-time is only compelled to spend twenty-six hours a week in patient-related activities, and that twenty-six hours can include travelling to and from patients' houses.

The average GP will do a morning surgery of one to two hours from Monday to Friday, and then be available for routine visits for a further hour. He will do an afternoon surgery of one to two hours on perhaps three afternoons a week. He has two afternoons a week off.

His on-call, including Saturday morning work, is likely to be shared in a rota with partners or other doctors. He will take at least six weeks holiday a year, maybe more.

Most GPs are bad time-managers and appalling business men. They think they are working long hours. It is not true. They are probably organising their work very badly, but in conventional terms they are not overworked.

If they hand over their on-call to a deputising service, and more than fifty per cent of them do, they may only work a thirty-hour week.

But the job has become unacceptably stressful due to the obligation to provide instant medical care at all times, and more recently because of the avalanche of paperwork generated by new government regulations. The GP has reacted by categorising his time strictly into periods of 'on' and 'off' duty. Because the on-duty periods are so intolerable, the off-duty periods become extended and entrenched.

There is no country in the world other than the UK where a patient can summon a doctor to his bedside at any time of the day or night for any condition, however trivial. Although the doctor is not obliged to visit, if he declines to do so inappropriately he will be held legally responsible for the consequences. The definition of "appropriate" or "inappropriate" in this context is determined retrospectively by an independent tribunal. Is it realistic to expect a doctor to get out of bed at three o'clock in the morning to visit a four-year old with a temperature? Such calls are commonplace. If the doctor declines to visit and the child later turns out to have meningitis, he may be sued.

In practice, the GP can never decline to see an insistent patient. However busy he is, however many patients are waiting to see him, if someone telephones and says they need to be seen urgently they have to be squeezed in immediately. The patient's definition of urgent is a loose one. "I just need something to throw of this head cold. I'm going on holiday on Saturday." Most doctors – indeed most sane people – would not regard this as an urgent medical problem. But the week before a Bank Holiday twenty or thirty such patients will demand immediate attention, and most of them will sulk when the doctor declines to prescribe an inappropriate antibiotic.

Junior Hospital Doctors

All junior doctors will one day apply to become consultants or GPs. To do this they will have to get good references from those lucky enough to be consultants or GPs already. To obtain a good reference, the nose must either be clean, or, even better, brown.

Above all else, they must not be known as trouble-makers.

The astute junior soon realises that all GPs and consultants look through rose-coloured spectacles at the years they spent in the hospital service. As they remember it, the Dunkirk spirit saw them through and they did not whinge. So why should the juniors be whingeing now? It must be the trouble-makers.

The basic contracted working week for junior hospital doctors is forty hours. But even in the quietest of specialities, like dermatology, more hours will be required. These will be unpaid. On top of that there is the on-call commitment.

"When I was a lad . . ."

Junior hospital doctors refer to their jobs as 1-in-2's, or 1-in-3's or 1-in-4's and so on. A 1-in-2 job involves working every other night and every other weekend. The weekend starts at 5.00 pm on the Friday evening and finishes at 9.00 am on Monday morning, a total of sixty-four hours. The doctor must get through a further routine eight hours of the Monday making a total stretch of seventy-two hours. In the busy specialities there really may have been no sleep at all during that period, unless one counts catnaps in Casualty over a snatched cup of coffee. 'Routine' work on a Monday morning may mean a busy operating list. Do you want your hip replaced by a doctor who has not slept for sixty-four hours?

Monday night is then free. But the next shift starts sixteen hours later at 9.00 am on Tuesday and continues through to 5.00 pm on Wednesday – a further thirty-two hours. Finally, there is 9.00 am Thursday morning through till 5.00 pm Friday, another thirty-two. The grand total for the week is thus one hundred and thirty-six hours.

The New Regime

1-in-2 jobs were once the norm. They have now been banned. No junior is supposed to be asked to work more than a 1-in-3 rota i.e. the normal working week plus every *third* night and every *third* weekend.

Trust hospitals, ever keen to save a penny, will compel juniors to cross-cover each others' holidays; this avoids additional expenditure on locums, but means that the junior notionally working a 1-in-3 is back to the good old 1-in-2. Such arrangements are forbidden, but if the junior never complains, no-one will ever know.

Wise and ambitious juniors do not complain. They put up with the long hours, knowing that one day their turn will come. It is all part of medical machismo. And above all, they dare not risk offending the boss. After all, he had to do it, as he never tires of telling them.

So will the boss allow his junior doctors any time off at all? That depends on his qualifications. Is he an MD or an MD? Confused? Yes, it can be difficult to tell. MD means either 'Doctor of Medicine' or 'Medical Dinosaur'. Juniors working for the latter kind of consultant have to be careful, or they will not get a reference.

There are a hundred and sixty-eight hours in a week. Of what activities, other than patient care, do the dinosaurs approve? In the table below are time allocations for allowable non-medical activities.

Time Allocation for Essential Non-Medical Activities

Activity	Minutes per day	Minutes per week	Weekly Total
Eating	90	630	10 hours 30 minutes
Bath/shower/teeth	30	210	2 hours 30 minutes
Lavatory	10	70	1 hour 10 minutes
Dressing/undressing	15	105	1 hour 45 minutes
Total	**145**	**1,015**	**15 hours 55 minutes**

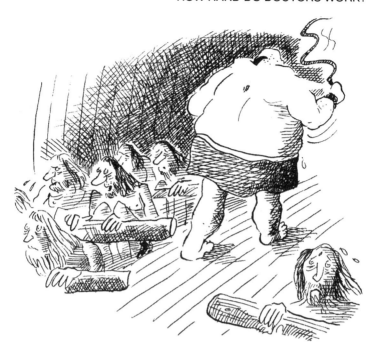

"Cheer up! We could have been Junior Doctors."

Some consultants would consider these allocations over-generous. Beer is one of the great colonic lubricators and so it is extravagant, they would argue, to allow over an hour a week to evacuate the organ. On the other hand, women need the time as they do not regularly consume vats of beer. Then again, medical dinosaurs do not recognise the existence of women doctors.

After taking away the fifteen hours fifty-five minutes of allowable non-medical activities, there are about a hundred and fifty-two hours left for patient care. The dinosaurs may sanction time off for golf, rugger or goat-shagging, but not for wimpish activities like sleep, illness or study.

There have been some improvements in the treatment of junior doc-

tors over the last ten years. The regulations now state that from April 1993 no junior doctor should be required to be on duty for more than an average of eighty-three hours a week if working an on-call rota. From January 1995 this will be reduced to seventy-two hours a week.

Regulations are designed for circumvention and there are many ways for hospitals to get round these restrictions. Until juniors have the whole-hearted support of their senior colleagues they will be risking career advancement every time they complain. Thus, even with the new regulations, anyone going into medicine still faces the prospect of spending many of the best years of their lives working long hours in hospitals for a poor financial reward.

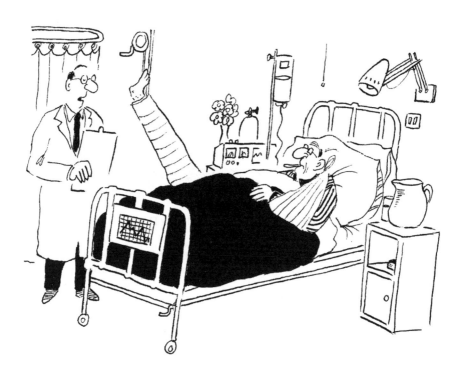

"Don't worry, we'll have you up and out of here in no time. The hospital's closing down on Monday."

THE PATIENT'S GUIDE TO HOSPITAL DOCTORS

Introduction

Categorising the medical profession used to be so easy: surgeons cut things out; obstetricians pulled things out; and physicians did everything else. But the pitch has been muddied by a plethora of specialities and sub-specialities which have sprung up, and which are no respecters of traditional professional boundaries.

This has put a strain on intra-professional relations. Hospital doctors behave territorially, like wild animals. The successful specialist not only knows his own territory; he also does his utmost to make sure other groups don't invade it. But he is not always successful. In times of change there are losers as well as winners.

The **general surgeons** and the **general physicians** are the losers. They used to have the largest areas and therefore the greatest kudos. But their areas were so large that they have been unable to defend them successfully from marauding sub-specialists. The kudos remains for the present, but will disappear when patients realise they have no territory left they can call their own.

Similar tensions affect all the other specialities, some on the up, some on the down.We will consider them in three groups. The *surgeons*, the *physicians* and the *rest*.

For each we will provide a consumer summary mentioning the following attributes:

1. Length of training

2. Private income potential

3. Probability of Merit Award

4. Whether the speciality is coming or going

5. Medical Machismo rating

To calibrate medical machismo we need some standard guidelines. The ultimate speciality for the tough guys, the Ruperts of the medical world, is cardiac surgery. This has a medical machismo rating of one hundred percent. At the other end of the scale we have non-hospital appointments. They hardly register and so are not included in the tables.

The lowly GP would score one or two percent. Not nought mind you. That accolade is reserved for the community physicians. Whoever they are.

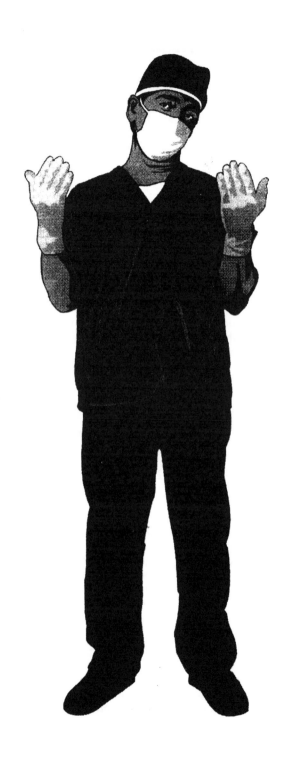

THE SURGEONS

Training for surgery is long and arduous, with a high drop-out rate along the way. An FRCS is essential. An MD or MS is helpful but optional. Most doctors think surgeons are arrogant shits. This is unfair; only some are. Surgeons are doers not thinkers. They are proud of their barber origins. If a patient has a medical problem that requires thought rather than excision, they refer the patient to the physicians. "Get the *doctors* to see him" they will tell the registrar.

Accident & Emergency Surgeons

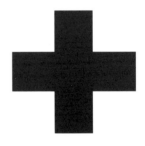

In the USA, traumatology has become one of the most exciting areas of medicine. The technology and expertise concentrated in American traumatology units means that patients involved in major road traffic accidents and the like are surviving horrific injuries.

The figures for survival from similar injuries in this country do not compare well. They are appalling. British accident and emergency departments have traditionally been staffed by inexperienced SHOs with no consultant back-up. The departments are under the notional control of one of the other specialists, usually the orthopaedic surgeons, whose main interests are elsewhere.

Recently, half-hearted and characteristically under-funded efforts have been made to attract consultants to a new and defined speciality of Accident & Emergency medicine. Where consultants have been appointed they usually have to work on their own without a consultant colleague to share the cover. They are unlikely to have any experienced junior staff above the level of SHO.

A vicious circle has been established. The work is hard, under-funded and monotonous. There is no opportunity for private practice. The mainstream specialists such as the general surgeons and physicians do not acknowledge the validity of the speciality. When the hospital is on stand-by for a major emergency (a 'red-alert'), they come in and take over. In the USA the traumatology department would be co-ordinating the whole show and have overall charge.

Because the speciality is not respected nor taken seriously, it does not attract high-fliers; without high-fliers, it remains a medical backwater. It is a home for failed orthopaedic surgeons, and doctors who have hit the brick wall of discrimination.

This not only damages a fledgling and deserving speciality but also damages the hospital. A hospital without a good A & E department withers because it is not at the front end of medicine.

To compound matters, the government is trying to close down Accident & Emergency departments because they are expensive.

Accident & Emergency Surgery

Summary	*For:* nothing *Against:* dead-end job – not real surgery
Length of Training	Uncertain. Specialist training now being introduced.
Private Income potential	Very poor indeed, apart from medico-legal reports
Probability of Merit Award	Hopeless
Coming or going	Has potential – when traumatology is recognised in the UK
Medical Machismo rating	10% 20% 30% 40% 50% 60% 70% 90% 90% 100%

Cardiac Surgeons

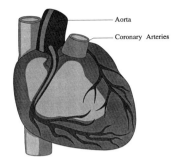

Aorta

Coronary Arteries

Cardiac and thoracic surgeons start off doing the same training. At senior registrar level they begin to sub-specialise in either heart or lung surgery. The heart or cardiac surgeon is considered the more glamorous of the two.

The hospital training is horrific. The surgeon must first do general surgical training and get an FRCS. At middle-grade registrar level he goes back to SHO level and starts again in cardio-thoracic. The hours are interminable. Until the recent change in regulations it could be a 1-in-2 rota for ten years. Even at senior registrar level it was probably a 1-in-2 because no other surgical speciality can cross-cover. The divorce rate is high. The second wife is frequently a Sister from one of the cardio-thoracic wards. She understands what is going on.

The cardiac surgeon is a man's man. This is 'the business'. He does not suffer fools – defined as those who don't agree with him – gladly. He treats his junior staff appallingly. He doesn't give a damn about merit awards, though he probably has one, because he is earning so much in the private sector.

Cardiac Surgery	
Summary	*For:* unsurpassed wealth & kudos *Against:* failed marriage, arrogance
Length of Training	10-15 years
Private Income potential	Huge: £500,000 is possible
Probability of Merit Award	Good, but irrelevant because their private income is vast
Coming or going	Has arrived and is staying
Medical Machismo rating	10% 20% 30% 40% 50% 60% 70% 90% 90% **100%**

General Surgeons

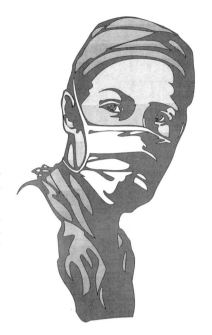

*"A fashionable surgeon like a
pelican can be recognised by the
size of his bill."*

J. CHALMERS DA COSTA (1863-1933)

There is a certain breed of surgeon who
genuinely though falsely believes that he
can maintain sufficient expertise to perform any operation. These true general
surgeons, ones that will "have a go" at
anything, should no longer exist. They
are Lancelot Spratts. They love operating. They circle round the patient like
Battle of Britain pilots, suddenly shout,
"O.K. Chaps, we're going in", and the

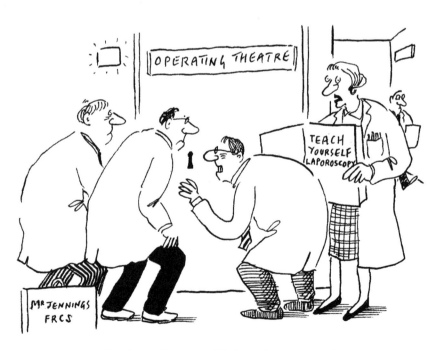

"So that's why they call it keyhole surgery . . ."

General Surgery

Summary	*For:* great history and tradition *Against:* Jack of all Trades – the surgical GP
Length of Training	10+ years
Private Income potential	Huge: .£200,000
Probability of Merit Award	Reasonable
Coming or going	Being eclipsed by sub-specialities
Medical Machismo rating	10% 20% 30% 40% 50% **60%** 70% 90% 90% 100%

unfortunate patient is whisked off to the operating theatre. They have become Jack of all Trades; their business cards read 'No job too small.'

If the general surgeons are anything at all, they are gut surgeons; abdominal surgeons. They repair herniae; they remove bowel blockages, malignant and benign. They also strip varicose veins; and a bit of this and a bit of that. They need a sub-speciality and so have with great joy grabbed the laporoscopc from the gynaecologists to perform so called 'keyhole surgery'.

Keyhole surgery is a great technological development, and in the right hands is safe, effective, cost-cutting and complication-avoiding. The old fashioned open operation to remove a gall-bladder meant a large abdominal incision and a week to ten days in hospital. Performed by laporoscope, there is a minute incision and the patient can go home the same day. Provided the operation is not cocked up.

And here lies the problem. There have been no specific training programmes for laporoscopic surgery, and far too many general surgeons have just decided to have a go and teach themselves, with unpleasant, sometimes catastrophic, results for the patient.

Still, there is lots and lots of private money in general surgery, provided you keep the GPs sweet.

Gynaecological Surgeons

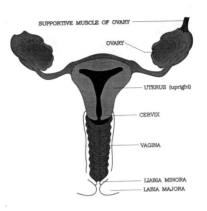

SUPPORTIVE MUSCLE OF OVARY

OVARY

UTERUS (upright)

CERVIX

VAGINA

LABIA MINORA
LABIA MAJORA

"The difference between a gynaecologist and a dentist is the angle of the chair."

ANON

Consultant obstetricians and gynaecologists are characteristically rich, smarmy misogynists. In temperament and attitude they are the nearest any group of doctors gets to madwives. Which is perhaps not surprising, because they spend the whole of their working life with them. Gynaecologists insist on being called "Mister". The surgeons, or 'real' surgeons as they see themselves in this context, regard the gynaecologists as surgical amateurs. Woe betide the gynaecologist who strays outside the pelvis and dares to, for example, take out an appendix. If anything goes wrong, his general surgical colleagues will crucify him.

Gynaecology involves looking after women's problems and is therefore regarded by other doctors as a speciality best reserved for women. Male doctors going into it used to have negative medical machismo. But an interesting transformation is taking place in the relationship between gynaecologists and their colleagues. For years the gynaecologists have been doing laporoscopic surgery. This is better known as keyhole surgery. Recently the general surgeons, ever keen to enlarge their shrinking patch, have realised that they could take out gall bladders through laporoscopes. "After all, it must be easy. The bloody gynaecologists do it."

It is not easy. When the general surgeons started borrowing the gynaecologists' laporoscopes there was a catalogue of well-publicised disasters. What effect has this had? Firstly, a public outcry about general surgeons arrogantly assuming they can start using new techniques without training. *See one, do one, teach one* may be all right for students, but not for surgeons. Secondly, an increase into double figures for the gynaecologists' machismo rating as their colleagues realised they can at least do one clever operation.

Why does anyone go into gynaecology? Not to pursue an interest in obstetrics. As the doctor progresses up the hierarchy, the more senior he gets, the fewer babies he delivers. When he becomes a consultant, his deliveries will be restricted to the odd private patient, the wives and daughters of colleagues, and the occasional difficult delivery when the registrar is otherwise tied up. The older a consultant is, the rustier his obstetric abilities become. He still does ante-natal clinics but is a stranger in the delivery suite.

The consultant obstetrician and gynaecologist spends over ninety per cent of his time doing gynaecology, and most gynaecology involves dealing with women with irregular periods.

The mainstay of gynaecological surgery is the D & C. This stands for *dilation* and *curettage*. It is generally known as a 'scrape' which describes the procedure well. The customer thinks it is a curative procedure for all period problems. It is not. It is purely a diagnostic procedure to check that the lining of the womb is normal, and, in particular, to exclude malignancy. Thousands of women have it done every year. Whatever purpose it may serve in theory, in practice it often *is* curative. Whether it is the psychological effect of seeing a gynaecologist, or the trauma of having an operation, or the reassurance of knowing that there is no underlying malignancy, patients who have presented with painful or irregular periods do not seem to return after a D & C. A D&C takes ten minutes. A consultant could do ten D&C's on Saturday morning at the private clinic and still take his dog for a walk before lunch.

The gynaecologist's favourite procedure is the hysterectomy. This operation is done far too often, particularly in America, but also in middle-class, privately-insured Britain. Hence, 'Wombless Woking'.

Gynaecological Surgery

Summary	*For:* always in demand *Against:* have to work with madwives
Length of Training	8-10 years
Private Income potential	Huge: >£250,000
Probability of Merit Award	Average
Coming or going	Entrenched
Medical Machismo rating	10% 20% **35%** 50% 60% 70% 90% 90% 100%

Neurosurgeons

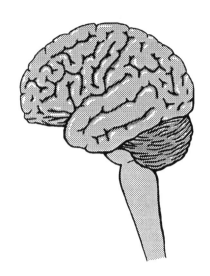

Brain surgery has a certain music hall comedy ethos. One imagines E.L. Gumbey being a brain surgeon, and indeed some of them do rather resemble him.

Brain surgery is not a popular speciality. It is boring. Operating on brains is like operating on a bowl of yesterday's muesli. It requires academic and surgical skills, which is an odd and unhappy combination.

Neorosurgery	
Summary	*For:* the layman is impressed *Against:* re-arranging cereal
Length of Training	10+ years
Private Income potential	£100,000
Probability of Merit Award	Reasonable
Coming or going	Here to stay
Medical Machismo rating	10% 20% 35% **40%** 50% 60% 70% 90% 90% 100%

Ophthalmic Surgeons

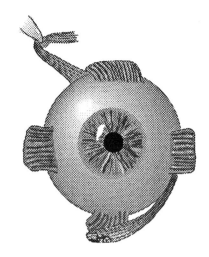

Everyone is squeamish about eyes. The idea of operating on them makes us squirm. Medical students are no different and not many start off wanting to go into ophthalmology, or "eyes" as it is more simply called.

This is a mistake, because it is a well-paid speciality with few out-of-hours problems. It is an almost completely circumscribed speciality. Contact with other doctors, other than diabetologists, is rare.

The routine work is cataracts, more cataracts and yet more cataracts. Possibly because no one else understands eyes, eye doctors are respected. They are very rich, and have the free time to spend their money.

Ophthalmology	
Summary	*For:* well-paid and interesting *Against:* not a lot
Length of Training	up to 10 years
Private Income potential	Excellent: £200,000
Probability of Merit Award	Reasonable
Coming or going	Here to stay
Medical Machismo rating	10% 20% 30% 40% **55%** 70% 90% 90% 100%

Orthopaedic Surgeons

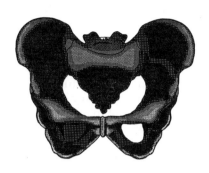

The classical bone doctor, or orthopod, is a big, hairy rugger-bugger. His medical machismo rating is lower than might be expected because his colleagues regard him as decerebrate. Orthopaedics certainly requires strength, but some women have succeeded in it in spite of that.

The orthopods like to call themselves traumatologists. They are facing a political fight as to who should be running the hospital when there is a disaster. So far, they have seen off the Accident & Emergency surgeons, but the real battle is yet to be won. Once the appalling record of traumatology in this country becomes public knowledge, there will be a shake-up. In the meantime, the increasing and never-ending stream of trauma makes this a busy and growing speciality. There is excellent scope for private practice, and articulate orthopods - rare beasts - make a fortune writing medico-legal reports.

Orthopaedic Surgery

Summary	*For:* a large and growing speciality *Against:* beware the A&E surgeons
Length of Training	10 years
Private Income potential	> £200,000
Probability of Merit Award	Reasonable
Coming or going	Ever-expanding
Medical Machismo rating	10% 20% 30% 40% **50%** 60% 70% 90% 90% 100%

Plastic Surgeons

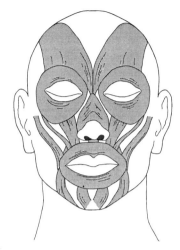

Beware the *'cosmetic* surgeon'. He is the one who advertises in the papers. "New boobs for old". He preys on human frailty and offers expensive surgical procedures for psychological problems. He is unlikely to be properly trained. He may not even have an FRCS. He certainly does not hold a health service consultant appointment, or he would not be doing the job he is doing.

The true plastic surgeons have an FRCS and have gone all the way up the medical hierarchy to consultant level. Their main work is re-constructive operations after major burns, cancer surgery and trauma. They have a reputation for being unwilling do to purely cosmetic procedures. This is

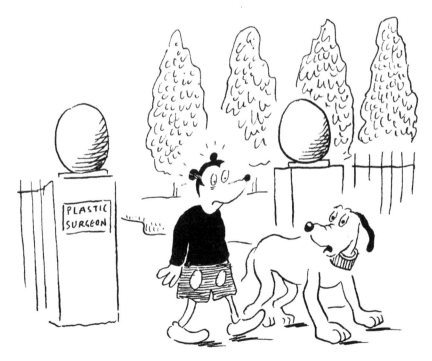

"But big ears *suited* you."

unfounded. They will do cosmetic surgery, although rarely on the NHS these days.

Face lifts, nose jobs, breast enlargement and reduction and many other cosmetic procedures can all be done by the plastic surgeon. But they will be done honestly. They will tell you that they cannot make you look forty years younger. Nor can they make fat people thin.

They will not operate on patients who are psychologically unstable; they will not promise the impossible; they will show you before and after photographs of the kind of results they can achieve; if there are post-operative problems, they will do their best to sort them out.

The plastic surgeon's income depends on his willingness, ability and opportunity to do cosmetic surgery. The potential is vast.

Plastic Surgery

Summary	*For:* can be very satisfying *Against:* few posts, difficult to get consultancy
Length of Training	10 years
Private Income potential	The sky's the limit with a large cosmetic private practice
Probability of Merit Award	Poor
Coming or going	Small but well-established
Medical Machismo rating	10% 20% 30% 45% 60% 70% 90% 90% 100%

Thoracic Surgeons

These are the guys who do the same initial training as the cardiac surgeons but who, for reasons known best to themselves, branch off into lungs. They tend to have a chip on their shoulder that they are not doing the glamorous stuff i.e. heart transplants. Their training is just as arduous as their cardiac colleagues but the status is not the same.

Nor is the money.

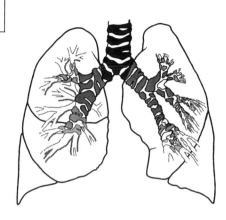

Thoracic Surgery	
Summary	*For:* well-paid *Against:* rather boring
Length of Training	10-15 years
Private Income potential	reasonable: >£100,000
Probability of Merit Award	Reasonable
Coming or going	Here to stay
Medical Machismo rating	10% 20% 30% 45% 50% 60% **70%** 90% 90% 100%

Urological Surgeons

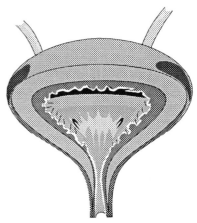

Urological surgeons specialise in kidneys, bladders, prostates, genitalia and incontinence. Much of their time is spent sitting between the legs of the patient looking down a cystoscope – a tubular metal instrument that can be stuck through a urethra into the patient's bladder.

The most common operation is a trans-urethral resection of prostate glands and bladder cancers. With a rapidly ageing population there is lots of demand for their services and trained urologists are in short supply. Many elderly men don't get their prostate looked at until their bladders are blocked and then the operation has to be done as an emergency. Urological surgeons work hard and are rich.

Urology	
Summary	*For:* money *Against:* working life spent looking down willies
Length of Training	10 years
Private Income potential	> £300,000
Probability of Merit Award	Good
Coming or going	Rapidly expanding
Medical Machismo rating	10% 20% 30% 45% **55%** 60% 70% 90% 90% 100%

Vascular Surgeons

The surgical equivalent of Dyn-a-Rod. The vascular surgeon is a plumber, although not as well paid. He unblocks or replaces clogged-up arteries.

This is yet another area that has been stolen from the general surgeons. The sub-speciality of vascular surgery is recent and is gaining ground quickly. Everyone knows that the coronary arteries get blocked with cholesterol; few realise that exactly the same process can happen to any artery in the body.

Most general surgeons have to do some vascular work, because when it is their night on-call, they will be covering for ruptured aortic aneurysms. The aorta is the main artery in the body. It comes out of the heart and runs down to the lower abdomen where it divides to supply blood to the legs. If this blood vessel ruptures, only immediate surgery will save the patient's life. It is a difficult and dangerous procedure, best done by vascular specialists. In the UK it is usually done by whichever surgeon happens to be around. The wise patient checks the surgical on-call rota at the local hospital and ruptures his aneurysm only if the vascular team is on duty.

Vascular Surgery	
Summary	*For:* ability to cure patients *Against:* not much
Length of Training	10 years
Private Income potential	>£200,000
Probability of Merit Award	Reasonable
Coming or going	Well-established and growing
Medical Machismo rating	10% 20% 30% 45% **55%** 60% 70% 90% 90% 100%

THE PHYSICIANS

"Doctors are men who prescribe medicine of which they know little to cure diseases of which they know less in human beings of which they know nothing."

VOLTAIRE (1694-1778)

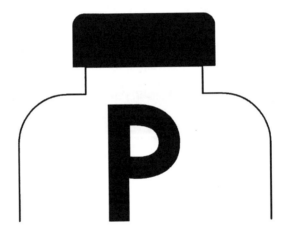

Surgeons examine patients and cut something out. Physicians, or "the doctors" as the surgeons call them, examine patients and prescribe tablets. Physicians are pill-pushers. Sophisticated ones, maybe, but still pill-pushers.

If any doctors can be said to be intellectuals, it must be the physicians. They are nearly as grand as their surgical colleagues, and certainly as pompous. They have adjacent rooms on Harley Street, but are rarely as rich, unless they have some quasi-surgical procedure they can perform.

So who are the physicians, and what do they do?

Cardiologists

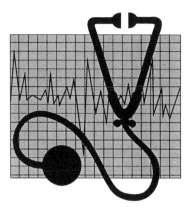

Cardiologists are respected by the layman, but they are fighting hard to avoid redundancy. Most of their traditional work is better done by machines or other doctors. Their territory is threatened. Nevertheless, they retain lots of medical machismo because they works with hearts, and hearts are glamorous.

The old style cardiologist was very clever indeed, or was perceived to be very clever, which is not quite the same thing. He was a master of the art of using the stethoscope. Heart murmurs are caused by blood passing through damaged heart valves or through abnormal communications between the four chambers of the heart. They are difficult to hear. They are even more difficult to analyse correctly and tie in with an anatomical diagnosis. The cardiologist listens with eyes closed, and then stands back from the bed to announce:

"Mitral regurgitation, aortic regurgitation and a deafening third heart sound."

Very impressive stuff too. Especially in the old days when there was no way of checking the validity of the diagnosis. Not that that mattered as there was nothing you could do about it anyway. Three great changes have spoiled the show:

1. Rheumatic fever and syphilis, the two most common causes of damage to heart valves, are now rare.

2. Imaging techniques such as echocardiography, and CT and MR scanning have made it possible to get a precise anatomical diagnosis of structural heart problems.

3. The heart can now be by-passed making open-heart surgery possible.

The cardiological emperor has been caught without his clothes. His clinical diagnosis of structural cardiac defects was often wrong. Cardiac surgeons can now repair or replace damaged valves and correct many of the other structural abnormalities but will not open a chest until they have a confirmed diagnosis. This is provided accurately by an echocardiogram – a machine. The cardiologist's best guess as to the diagnosis is ignored; unless it is wrong, in which case the cardiac surgeon takes the piss.

Cardiology	
Summary	*For:* glamour and machismo *Against:* is it a valid job any more?
Length of Training	> 10 years
Private Income potential	£100,000
Probability of Merit Award	Good
Coming or going	Could be taken over by other specialities. Wait until Mrs Bottomley hears
Medical Machismo rating	10% 20% 30% 45% 50% 60% **75%** 90% 100%

So what is left for the cardiologist? Not a lot without elbowing into other doctors' territory. Patients with angina are referred to cardiologists for a treadmill test. The patient is attached to an ECG machine and exercised to see if there are changes suggestive of blockage of the coronary arteries. This test can be done by a technician and a machine. It *is* done by a technician and a machine, notionally supervised by the cardiologist.

Next, the cardiologist does an angiogram. This involves passing a cannula from the femoral artery in the groin right up the body to the heart and then injecting dye. An X-ray picture will then show any blockages in the coronary arteries. Sometimes these blockages can be dilated there and then (angioplasty) but more usually the patient will be referred on to a cardio-thoracic surgeon for a Coronary Artery By-Pass Graft, known in the trade as a CABG (pronounced 'cabbage').

Arteriography and angioplasty are invasive techniques involving the reading and analysis of complicated X-rays. The job would be better done by radiologists who have specialised training in these fields. The cardiologists strenuously deny this, but then they would, wouldn't they? If they didn't have angiograms to do, they'd be out of a job.

Glamour keeps the punter interested in private referrals, but for how long?

Chest Physicians

"Cure for consumption: Cut up a little turf of fresh earth and laying down breathe into the hole a quarter of an hour... In the last stage suck a healthy woman. This cured my father."
JOHN WESLEY (1703-91) PRIMITIVE PHYSIC

This used to be a dead-end job. The old chest physicians looked after TB sanatoria. There was no treatment for TB other than isolation and fresh air, so the job was administrative. Don't knock it. If it hadn't been for the sanatoria, Galton and Simpson would never have met to write the Hancock and Steptoe scripts.

There were one or two rare but interesting conditions for them to diagnose, such as pigeon fanciers lung, but it was all academic nonsense as there was no treatment they could offer having made the diagnosis.

The advent of effective treatment for asthma, and heavy smokers in the Royal Family, have combined to revitalise the job. It is again a respected speciality.

Chest Medicine	
Summary	*For:* Treating asthma is rewarding *Against:* Difficult to get into
Length of Training (years)	< 10 years
Private Income potential	>£50,000
Probability of Merit Award	Average to good
Coming or going	Well-established but static
Medical Machismo rating	10% 20% 30% 45% **55%** 70% 80% 90% 100%

Dermatologists

If a doctor wants a good private income and a quiet life, this is the place to be. Dermatology patients never get better, never die, and never call you out at night.

The GP diagnoses a rash which he describes as an odd, erratically-shaped, red patch. The dermatologist translates the description into Latin, puts a serious look on his face, tells the patient that he has *erythema multiforme* and collects £60 from BUPA. Nice work if you can get it.

If the dermatologist does not know which Latin words to use, he chops a bit of the rash out and sends it to a pathologist who will look at it under a microscope and make the diagnosis for him. He has a larger Latin dictionary. It's as easy as that.

Dermatology	
Summary	*For:* a quiet life *Against:* gob-stoppingly dull
Length of Training	8 years
Private Income potential	£50,000
Probability of Merit Award	Poor to average
Coming or going	Like itching, just will not go away
Medical Machismo rating	15% 30% 45% 50% 60% 70% 80% 90% 100%

Diabetologists

"In a case of suspected diabetes you must examine the urine," the professor told the medical students. "Dip the finger in and taste the sugar" he said and proceeded to demonstrate. The specimen bottle was then passed around the students who repeated the test with varying degrees of disgust.

"Now, ladies and gentlemen. Notice that I dipped in my index finger and sucked my ring finger. In medicine observation is crucial."

APOCRYPHAL

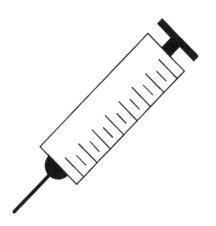

Looking after diabetes is important work.

It is also dull, boring and repetitive. Routine diabetic care is best done by the experts in dull, boring and repetitive work: nurses. It is what they are trained for. The best diabetic clinics have a team of diabetic liaison nurses who provide an outstanding service.

Hospital diabetic follow-up clinics are awful. The consultants do not go near them. They are staffed by the most junior of junior hospital doctors who change every six months just before they begin to understand what they are doing. The patient attending the clinic is kept waiting as long as possible. By the time he is called into the consulting room he has learnt his copy of the Citizens Charter off by heart. The young doctor flips helplessly through the invariably large set of notes, calls the patient by the wrong name, and then, if he finds the latest blood tests, tells him off for not controlling his diabetes properly. Diabetics hate going to the hospital clinics.

Many GPs are frightened of diabetics. They are too far away from their hospital jobs to remember how to manipulate insulin doses and so rely on the nursing liaison sister for advice. Doctors are not good at taking advice from nurses.

Switched-on GPs run their own diabetic clinics at the health centre. These provide a better standard of care than the average hospital clinic staffed by juniors.

94

Diabetologists are a threatened species. There has already been some success with pancreatic transplants and it is only a matter of time before the condition is effectively curable.

Not much private practice as no 'procedure' to perform.

Diabetology	
Summary	*For:* important job at present *Against:* boring
Length of Training	8-10 years
Private Income potential	> £20,000
Probability of Merit Award	Good
Coming or going	Will disappear soon when pancreatic transplants are sorted out
Medical Machismo rating	10% 20% **35%** 50% 60% 70% 80% 90% 100%

Endocrinologists

"It's my glands, doctor."

The perpetual cry of the obese middle-aged woman. It rarely *is* her glands, but if it is, she will be looked after by an endocrinologist. They deal with the sweetbreads: thyroids, pancreases, adrenals, parathryroids, the lot. This is complicated and clever medicine that most other doctors do not understand.

Endocrinologists will be threatened by a large number of unemployed diabetologists when pancreas transplants arrive in force.

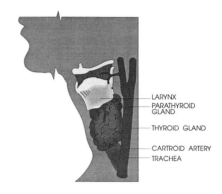

LARYNX
PARATHYROID GLAND
THYROID GLAND
CARTROID ARTERY
TRACHEA

Endocrinology	
Summary	*For:* clever stuff *Against:* small-print stuff
Length of Training	> 10 years
Private Income potential	> £20,000
Probability of Merit Award	Average
Coming or going	A minority interest
Medical Machismo rating	10% 20% **35%** 50% 60% 70% 80% 90% 100%

Gastroenterologists

Most people do not realise that their gut is one long, tortuous tube that goes from the back of the throat to the anus. The gastroenterologist looks after it. What goes in. What comes out. The changes that take place in between. Diarrhoea is their bread and butter.

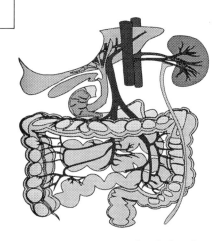

The liver works intimately with the gut, and so they look after that as well. They also look after the part of the pancreas that works on the gut, careful always not to impose upon the diabetologists who look after the part that makes the insulin.

Gastroenterology	
Summary	*For:* lucrative and interesting *Against:* a lot of shit
Length of Training	> 10 years
Private Income potential	> £120,000
Probability of Merit Award	Good
Coming or going	Well-established
Medical Machismo rating	10% 20% 30% 45% 50% **65%** 80% 90% 100%

Gastroenterologists are among the richer physicians because they have some practical procedures to perform, namely sticking tubes in the patients' tube: gastroscopies and colonoscopies (top and bottom).

They are in dispute with the general surgeons who believe that passing an endoscope into a patient's stomach is a skilled surgical procedure best done, naturally enough, by surgeons. The gastroenterologists acknowledge the surgeons' ability to pass a 'scope but are saddened that they do not have the intellect to recognise what they see down it.

The switched-on gastroenterologist can do half a dozen private-oscopies on a Saturday morning. The money is good.

General Physicians

'Nor bring to watch me cease to live
Some Doctor, full of phrase and fame
To shake his sapient head and give
The ill he cannot cure – a name'

MATTHEW ARNOLD (1822-88)

The eighteenth and nineteenth centuries were the age of the general physician. The universe of medical knowledge was small; sub-specialists were unnecessary; surgeons were not even recognised as members of the profession. General physicians rejoiced in their omniscience and omni-competence; they reigned supreme. As trained observers, they described and classified hitherto undefined conditions, rarely offering cures or even effective treatments. But doctors have an atavistic attitude to illness: their fear of the unknown evaporates when they can name a disease. Better for the patient to die of *Addison's* disease than adrenal failure.

The modern general physician has two problems: there are very few diseases left to be named and the twentieth century patient expects to be cured of his illness. A name will not suffice. Effective treatment of most illnesses now requires additional knowledge and the sub-specialist has taken over. General physicians may diagnose Addison's Disease, but it is best treated by the endocrinologists.

The general physicians have retaliated by 'taking an interest'. They style themselves as physicians "with an interest in . . . [cardiology], [gastroenterology], [whatever]." Well, not quite whatever; physicians do not have an interest in geriatrics, or if they do, they keep quiet about it.

There are rules about training and accreditation before an 'interest' can be declared, but the rules are flexible and predicated by hospital requirements. An interest may mean no more than what it says; indeed, it may only have developed when the doctor read the job advert. It would be dangerous to infer a high degree of sub-specialist training in the area of interest. The general physician with an interest in cardiology may not, for example, be trained to do angiography, and will refer patients needing that investigation to a cardiologist. Most of his hospital work will be caring for *crumble* until his junior staff can bounce it to the geriatricians.

Britain lost an Empire and could not find a role. The general physician is better off. His empire has gone, but he has a role. He is a geriatrician. All that remains is for him to acknowledge it.

General Physicians	
Summary	*For:* kudos *Against:* the bubble is about to burst
Length of Training	8-10 years
Private Income potential	Good at present but about to collapse
Probability of Merit Award	Good
Coming or going	Facing extinction
Medical Machismo rating	10% 20% 30% 45% 50% **65%** 80% 90% 100%

Geriatricians

Geriatricians look after patients who are beyond economic repair.

Hospital physicians do not like dealing with the elderly because they have an irritating habit of failing to respond to treatment and dying. All elderly patients are shunted off to geriatricians at the first opportunity.

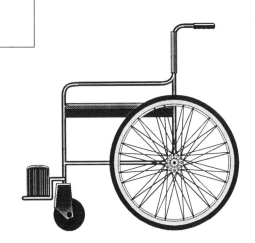

The reader should understand that the definition of 'elderly' in this context is highly specialised and depends on three factors:

Chronological age

The doctor's interest starts to wane as the patient passes sixty-five. After seventy-five medical treatment is regarded as a bit of a waste of time and after eighty-five it is seen to be contra-indicated.

The medical condition from which the patient suffers

Strokes,dementia, Parkinson's disease etc. are all a big turn-off. Patients with these sorts of problem are deemed to be elderly however young they are.

The patient's ability to co-operate

Do not be difficult or stroppy with doctors. They punish unco-operative patients by handing them over to the geriatricians.

Junior hospital doctors call elderly patients 'crumble'.

A GP trying to arrange an acute hospital admission for a seventy-year-old who lives alone and has had a stroke will be met with a wall of indifference from the hospital registrar. "Can't the family cope?" or "Why don't you get the district nurses in?" or "We are very busy and this is a social problem really" is what he will hear.

Such is the physicians' indifference to the elderly that they have created a sub-species of doctor which they have called geriatricians. The geriatricians have MRCP but have fallen or have been pushed off the career ladder. They are allowed to pretend they are real physicians but are not treated as such.

There is a strong case for having physicians skilled in the needs of the elderly. It does not work like that. The medical registrars screen all the acute admissions. The geriatricians get the patients with chronic, incurable illnesses whatever their age. A fifty-five year old with a stroke will be put under the geriatricians. A seventy-five year old with an "interesting" cardiac arrhythmia will be kept by the general physicians.

Junior hospital doctors do not understand that ageing is a natural process; that no-one is exempt; that we have an ageing population; that everyone should be accorded a reasonable standard of medical care. They continue to talk about 'crumble' and continue to resist the admission of 'crumble' to their wards.

Fobbing off crumble is part of medical machismo. The registrar will sit at lunch and say, "That bloody GP wanted me to take some seventy-nine-year old crumble onto an acute medical ward. I ask you. Told him we were full." There will be murmurs of approval.

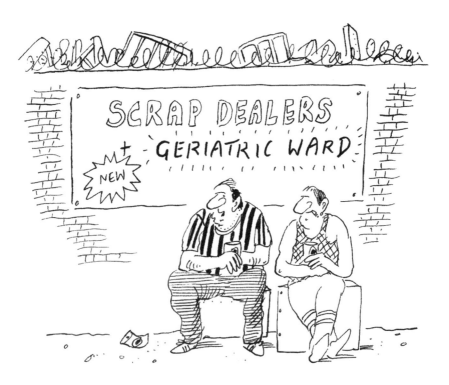

"We've got the premises, I thought to myself, so why not?"

Geriatrics	
Summary	*For:* rewarding job for the committed *Against:* treated with contempt by colleagues
Length of Training	7 years
Private Income potential	Nil. (Have you ever heard someone boasting about their private geriatrician?)
Probability of Merit Award	Very poor
Coming or going	All doctors will be geriatricians soon
Medical Machismo rating	5% 20% 30% 45% 50% 60% 70% 80% 90% 100%

The geriatrician is held in contempt by his colleagues. He is assumed to be a failed physician. Sadly, this assumption is usually fair. No medical student ever has an ambition to go into geriatrics.

Young doctors have a shock in store for them. When the post-war baby boomers reach seventy in the early part of the next century, all doctors will be geriatricians.

Nephrologists

Clever doctors, nephrologists. They specialise in kidney diseases, the failing kidney and kidney transplants. The transplant surgeons may get most of the glory but they are just technicians – mere plumbers. The clever stuff is keeping the patient alive until a transplant is ready, and then dealing with rejection afterwards.

Renal medicine is intensive and trendy.

A natural home for high fliers.

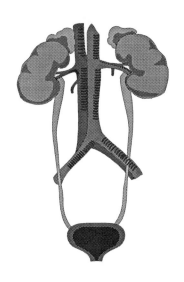

Nephrology	
Summary	*For:* trendy *Against:* intense competition for jobs
Length of Training	10 years
Private Income potential	> £50,000
Probability of Merit Award	Excellent
Coming or going	Fairly new but well-established
Medical Machismo rating	10% 20% 30% 45% 50% 60% **75%** 90% 100%

Neurologists

An academic and intellectual speciality. The neurologist uses inductive and deductive reasoning to tie up odd physical signs with rare diseases, and *vice versa*. Trouble is, once they have worked out what the diagnosis is, there is nothing they can do about it. Most neurological problems are incurable.

How to irritate a neurologist:

'The life expectancy of a patient with motor neurone disease is never more than five years; therefore Professor Stephen Hawking is a malingerer.'

Discuss.

Their day-to-day work is boring; tension headaches, migraine, and strokes. They have a similar problem to the cardiologists: their sophisticated clinical skills and diagnoses can now be checked by the CT scan. Nevertheless, they remain respected by their colleagues as "clever" doctors.

Neurology	
Summary	*For:* intellectually stimulating *Against:* can do nothing for their patients
Length of Training	10-15 years
Private Income potential	> £50,000
Probability of Merit Award	Good
Coming or going	Well-established
Medical Machismo rating	10% 20% 30% 45% 50% **60%** 70% 80% 90% 100%

Paediatricians

A once great speciality laid low by sub-specialists. The paediatrician is the general physician for children and will have an MRCP and probably an MD. Like his counterpart who deals with adults he has been unable to defend his territory and will soon be out of a job. Unlike his adult counterpart, he does not enjoy much kudos.

The problem with general paediatrics is that children only suffer from a small number of very serious diseases. These diseases are so serious and specialised that they are best treated in a teaching hospital, maybe even a specialised children's teaching hospital like Great Ormond Street in London or Alder Hey in Liverpool. These hospitals have a full range of sub-specialists such as paediatric cardiologists, paediatric nephrologists and so on. The general paediatrician in the district general hospital is not left much. A bit of asthma, a bit of this, a bit of that. Chronic constipation and bed-wetting will feature strongly, as will social deprivation. The consultant paediatrician has become more of a family therapist and social worker than a doctor. Grown-up doctors – doctors that treat grown-ups – are tolerant of and mildly amused by paediatricians but do not take them seriously.

Paediatrics	
Summary	*For:* patients are children *Against:* patients are children
Length of Training	10-12 years
Private Income potential	> £20,000
Probability of Merit Award	Below average
Coming or going	Well-established
Medical Machismo rating	10% **25%** 45% 50% 60% 70% 80% 90% 100%

Radiotherapists & Oncologists

Radiotherapists and oncologists look after patients with cancer. In many countries, these are two separate specialities.

There are very few pure medical oncologists in the UK, and they work mainly at cancer centres such as the Royal Marsden in London and the Christie in Manchester. They treat cancer patients with drugs or chemotherapy. They do not do operations. They do not themselves use radiotherapy. The chances of getting one of these consultancies are so small that few consider it. Those set on such a career, like media doc Rob Buckman, go abroad.

Oncologists	
Summary	*For:* rare and well-respected *Against:* impossible to get consultancy
Length of Training	> 10 years
Private Income potential	> £25,000
Probability of Merit Award	Very good
Coming or going	Has not yet arrived in UK
Medical Machismo rating	10% 20% 30% **48%** 60% 70% 80% 90% 100%

Radiotherapists are radiation physicians and, as their name suggests, treat cancer patients with radiotherapy. They also use chemotherapy. They think that medical oncology as a speciality is a waste of time because they can do the chemotherapy just as well. The oncologists dislike the way the radiotherapists "squirt a few drugs in". They particularly dislike the way radiotherapists insist on styling themselves as oncologists.

Radiotherapy is easy to get into. It is a home for both physicians and surgeons who have fallen off more competitive ladders. MRCP or FRCS is a common entrance exam. The radiotherapist with FRCS will revert to calling himself 'Doctor' rather than 'Mister'. Isn't it complicated?

General physicians treat oncologists with respect because they are rare. They treat radiotherapists like technicians. There is one consolation for all in this speciality: the rich may not get as much cancer as the poor, but there is enough about to provide lots of private practice.

Radiotherapy	
Summary	*For:* good money *Against:* treated like technicians
Length of Training	> 10 years
Private Income potential	> £50,000
Probability of Merit Award	Poor
Coming or going	A growth area
Medical Machismo rating	10% **20%** 30% 40% 50% 60% 70% 80% 90% 100%

Rheumatologists

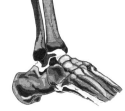

Rheumatologists specialise in 'physical' medicine. This means muscles, bones and joints – parts of the body that bore general physicians to death. Their most important work is dealing with Rheumatoid Arthritis. They also manage rare and unpleasant connective tissue diseases such as Systemic Lupus. Their routine clinics contain a rag bag of aches, pains and strains that the GPs have not been able to get rid of. Dreary work indeed. But lots of private practice. The rich and famous get lots of aches and pains.

Few doctors set out to be rheumatologists. Their interest arises as their career in general medicine flounders. They are poorly regarded by their colleagues, occupying a no-mans land between orthopaedic surgeons and general physicians. They are treated like up-market physiotherapists, which is what they are.

Rheumatology	
Summary	*For:* very little out-of-hours work *Against:* dull work for dull doctors
Length of Training	8 years
Private Income potential	> £50,000
Probability of Merit Award	Poor
Coming or going	Necessary
Medical Machismo rating	**15%** 30% 40% 50% 60% 70% 80% 90% 100%

Venereologists

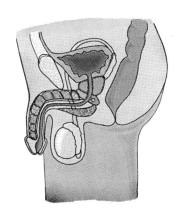

*'A night with Venus and a lifetime
with mercury'* [1]

TRADITIONAL

Well, would *you* want to do it?

The time taken to rise to consultant level in venereology is short. As
with all the unpopular jobs many of
the consultants are foreign. But some-
thing has happened. The Seven Knights of the **Serendip could** not have done
better than the consultants in what was traditionally the most unpopular
speciality of all. Along came AIDS, and with it an explosion of interest in
sexually-transmitted disease.

The general physicians have muscled in on the act but the venereologists,

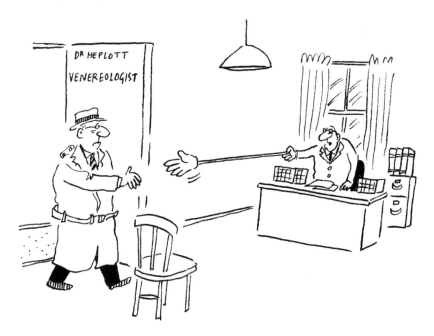

"Morning . ."

Venereology	
Summary	*For:* a speciality re-born *Against:* all the obvious things
Length of Training	6 years
Private Income potential	> £20,000
Probability of Merit Award	Poor
Coming or going	Coming +++
Medical Machismo rating	10% 20% 30% **40%** 50% 60% 70% 80% 90% 100%

or STD[2] physicians as they prefer to be called, have the background experience. HIV infection presents the medical profession with the greatest challenge it has faced this century, perhaps ever. It is now attracting the best brains of the profession.

Lots of private practice: the rich get sexually-transmitted diseases and are keen to have it treated discretely and privately.

1. A reference to the traditional treatment of syphilis with mercury It did not cure the disease and like many old-fashioned treatments was extremely unpleasant.

2. STD – Sexually Transmitted Diseases

THE REST

THE SERVICE INDUSTRIES

Most medical students say they are hoping for a career in general medicine or general surgery. At that stage in training any other career is something for the "also-rans". But the hard fact is that over 75% of students *will become* such "also-rans". Strangely, in view of the negative way it is still regarded by most teaching hospitals, some admit to an interest in general practice. Perhaps they are just the realistic ones.

Few, however, ever admit to an interest in the service industries: *radiology, pathology* and *haematology*. Many are not aware of their existence. Some say that they are not real medical specialities at all. As for psychiatry, those that do harbour ambitions in that direction will keep quiet about it if they do not want to be figures of fun throughout their training.

So what are the service industries all about, and who ends up in them?

Radiology
Pathology
Haematology
Psychiatry

The radiologists', pathologists' and haematologists' main role in life is to provide answers to questions asked by other doctors. With the exception of the haematologists, they have no direct relationship with the patient.

A much higher proportion of women are found at the top levels in these specialities. The training periods are shorter, the consultancies are easier to acquire and there is little out-of-hours responsibility. It is much easier to construct a career around childbirth.

Radiologists

In the old days, this was a dead-end job. The consultants often had no postgraduate qualifications other than a Diploma in Radiology. Clinicians still do not take radiologists too seriously. They think that any doctor can read an X-ray and that the radiologist is just a technician.

Science and technology has revolutionised the speciality. As well as ordinary X-ray machines there is now a range of highly sophisticated imaging equipment such as CT and MR scanners which enable the radiologist to make accurate anatomical diagnoses of medical pathology. It is this equipment which has undermined and made redundant the skills of the cardiologists and neurologists. The radiologists have developed techniques of cannulating arteries and veins which enable them to perform surgical operations without opening up the patient. The ultimate keyhole surgery.

The Royal College of Radiologists has encouraged the teaching hospitals to set up what amount to residency programmes in radiology. Registrars from medicine and surgery, and occasionally other specialities, are carefully

Radiology	
Summary	*For:* front line of technology *Against:* no patient contact
Length of Training	6 years
Private Income potential	> £75,000
Probability of Merit Award	Poor
Coming or going	Increasingly important
Medical Machismo rating	10% 20% **35%** 50% 60% 70% 80% 90% 100%

selected. They will already have a postgraduate qualification such as MRCP or FRCS. The number of entrants is balanced against the number of consultant posts likely to be available. The FRCR is maintained as a difficult exam and the second part is not taken until senior registrar level. It is an exit exam. Holders of FRCR know how to look at an X-ray.

Out-of-hours work has increased considerably with the advent of new technology but the commitment is still small. And there is lots of private practice to compensate.

Pathologists

There is a variety of sub-species of pathologist which we will discuss briefly, before giving a single classification of all but the Haematologists. They cannot quite decide whether they are clinicians or pathologists and keep a foot in both camps.

- **Microbiologists** look after bugs and bacteria. They are the snot, poo and wee-wee doctors. They analyse specimen of these and other bodily products to see what bacteria they contain. They advise on appropriate anti-biotics.

- **Chemical pathologists** analyse the same fluids for chemical content. A few of them run clinics and see live patients to advise on chemicals such as cholesterol and lipids.

- **Histopathologists** receive the bits and bobs the surgeons remove from patients and advise on tissue type and malignancies.

- **Forensic pathologists** are the ones everyone has heard of. Those who work for the Home Office follow the police around to pick up the remains of murder victims. The ordinary forensic pathologist spends most of his time performing autopsies on people who have been silly enough to die without giving due notice to the medical profession of their intentions.

Pathology is an academic subject. The training period is relatively short but FRCPath is one of the toughest exit exams and only the brightest candidates pass it first time. Some never get it. Passing the exam is almost a guarantee of a consultancy.

Private practice opportunities depend on the sub-speciality. The microbiologist and the chemical pathologist see very little unless they are exceptional entrepreneurs and set up their own private pathology clinics. Then the rewards can be enormous.

Histopathologists depend on the surgeons and dermatologists to send them specimens from their private patients. The decision as to which pathologist to use is at the whim of the surgeon. The wise histopathologist takes up goat-shagging at an early stage in his career.

Forensic pathologists have the best potential for a regular private income. They perform post-mortems for the coroner. This is not NHS work and so they are paid a separate fee, at present a stiff sixty six pounds, or sixty six pounds a stiff, whichever way you like it. They are likely to do one post-mortem a day, and it may be three or four. Some of them will slip a fiver to the mortuary technician leaving a net take before tax of over sixty pounds. Four hundred of these a year keeps them in beer.

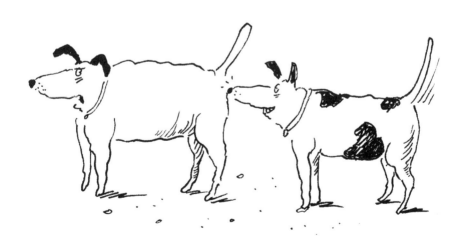

"Why's it always you who gets to be the microbiologist?"

Coroners' post mortems are not glamorous. They rarely involve foul play or medical cock-ups. They are usually just elderly people who have died unexpectedly. The unscrupulous pathologist will do the post-mortem in ten minutes. Opening up the skull is an essential part of the examination. But it is a messy, time-consuming business involving the use of a circular saw, and so is often omitted.

A plausible diagnosis of cause of death rather then an accurate one is what matters. If there is no question of foul play, no one is going to check.

Pathology	
Summary	*For:* appeals to the academic *Against:* messy and unpleasant work
Length of Training	> 6 years
Private Income potential	>£30,000 if doing coroner's work; very much less otherwise
Probability of Merit Award	Poor
Coming or going	Essential service
Medical Machismo rating	10% 25% 40% 50% 60% 75% 90% 100% Usually ..... but for famous Home Office pathologists

Haematologists

Haematologists are hybrid beasts. Unlike true pathologists, they cannot decide whether they prefer their patients dead or alive. They all have FRCPath but many have MRCP as well. Their laboratory work involves overseeing the technicians who process the requests for blood tests from the clinicians. Their own clinical work involves treating patients with blood disorders, such as leukaemia.

Private practice can be difficult. Their clinical colleagues cheat them out of work to keep costs down for the patient. Private patients should have private investigations. But it is very easy to keep a collection of NHS request forms in the brief case and quietly suggest to he patient that they go to the NHS hospital for their tests. This cheats the haematologist; it cheats the hospital; it cheats the NHS; it cheats the tax payer. It is fraud. It goes on all the time.

Haematologists are respected by their colleagues because they have mastered a difficult area of medicine that no one else understands and because they maintain clinical contact with patients.

Haematology	
Summary	*For:* combines academic and clinical *Against:* money not good
Length of Training	6 years
Private Income potential	> £15,000 - £20,000
Probability of Merit Award	Average
Coming or going	Static
Medical Machismo rating	10% 20% 30% **45%** 60% 70% 80% 90% 100%

Psychiatrists

• Are all psychiatrists mad?

Psychiatry is not a glamorous speciality. It is under-funded. It rarely attracts high-fliers, and those that do go into it rise quickly to the top. It is a job in which few students express an interest. There are many foreign doctors in psychiatry, some of whom do not speak good English.

Junior hospital doctors go into psychiatry either because they want to or because they cannot get a job in any other field. Of the ones who go into it through choice, most are mad; or peculiar; or both. Of the ones who are not mad or peculiar or both at the beginning of the training, most become so during it. The few that remain entirely normal become excellent psychiatrists.

• Community Care

The government is closing down the bins; or to quote from the manifesto, psychiatric care is becoming "community based". In essence, a laudable policy; in reality, because it is so lamentably under-funded, a disaster.

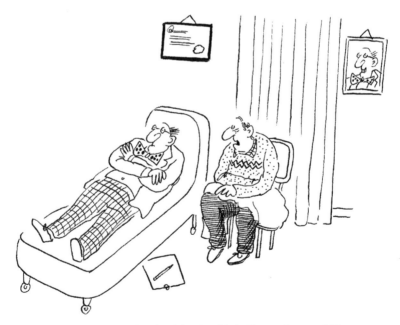

"Look, I'm paying for this, shouldn't *I* be on the couch?"

Psychiatry	
Summary	*For:* early retirement *Against:* treated as medical pariahs
Length of Training	8-10 years
Private Income potential	> £15,000
Probability of Merit Award	Poor
Coming or going	Static
Medical Machismo rating	7% 20% 30% 40% 50% 60% 70% 80% 90% 100%

Patients who desperately need on-going psychiatric care have been lost to the system. Before Margaret Thatcher the chronically mentally ill were called patients; now they are called tramps. The NHS does not even provide the cardboard boxes. This reduces the health care bill enormously.

Those doctors wishing to care for the cardboard box community have to pass MRCPschy. This is somewhere between an entrance and an exit exam. A few psychiatrists will also have taken an MRCP before they enter the speciality.

Psychiatrists have one great advantage over any other NHS employee. They can retire on full pension at fifty-five, provided they have been working for at least twenty years. This concession is an acknowledgement of the strains involved in looking after the mentally ill. It is nothing to do with the risk of becoming mentally ill. Allegedly.

Private practice opportunities should be reasonable, because the rich are just as likely to go potty as the poor. But most private health insurance excludes some or all of mental illness, and so earning potential is limited.

The best approach for avaricious psychiatrists is to found a private psychiatric clinic to care for media lushes.

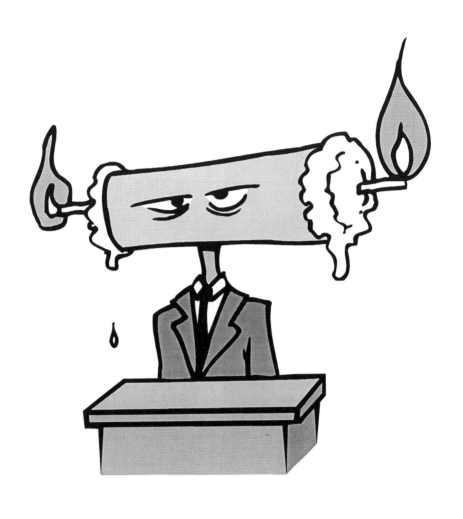

Burn Out

The Specialist Non-Specialist

Until fairly recently, there were no entry requirements for general practice, and no specific training or qualifications, other than the basic medical degree, were required. A newly-qualified doctor, having completed his two pre-registration jobs, could immediately enter general practice.

Doctors only went into general practice if they were unable to pursue a career in hospital medicine. It was the repository of failures, full either of those unable to get into consultant training or those who had fallen off the ladder during such training. Few self-respecting medical students would admit to a desire to go into general practice, and those who did would be regarded as lacking in ambition or as pre-ordained failures. Despite the fact that well over half the graduates would eventually go into general practice it was ignored as an intellectual discipline. Nothing was expected from GPs and so no training was provided.

There is a world of difference between hospital medicine and general practice. However experienced a hospital doctor may be, he will be lost during the first few weeks of general practice.

The majority of patients in hospital have identifiable, easily described organic pathology. They have already been screened by their GP, who has made the diagnosis and referred the patient to the appropriate speciality. The gynaecology registrar seeing a patient referred by the GP knows the problem will be gynaecological. In the unlikely event of it being a different problem, say for example a cardiac problem, the gynaecologist will simply refer the patient on to his cardiological colleague without giving the matter further thought.

Lack of Soap

The thought process drummed into the hospital doctor is described by the acronym S.O.A.P. Always think "soap". What does it mean? Nothing to do with cleanliness. The letters stand for:

- **Subjective**
    The patient's complaints, the history.

- **Objective**

  The physical findings, the examination.

- **Analysis**

  Conclusions & diagnosis

- **Plan**

  The action plan.

Plan has three important sub-headings:

- **Dx**

  Diagnostic tests

- **Rx**

  Treatment, either prescription or operation

- **Ex**

  Explanation

• Sx		Right upper hypochondrial pain aggravated by food
• Ox		Tender R hypochondrium Obese +++
• Ax		Gall stones
• Px	**Dx**	Ultrasound (already done by GP)
	Rx	Buscopan tablets for symptomatic relief til surgery
	Ex	Told to get some weight off

Let us consider a typical surgical registrar putting SOAP into action. We shall call him Rupert Spratt. Mrs B, an overweight, fading-blonde, middle-aged woman with three children has been referred to the hospital by her GP, Dr F, with recurrent abdominal pains and a diagnosis of gall stones. The registrar asks the patient if the pain is brought on by eating, which she confirms. He pops her up on the examination couch and prods her under the right ribs which makes her say "Ouch". He looks at the ultrasound test which the GP has already done which confirms the diagnosis of gall stones and books her in for an operation to remove her gall bladder. His notes will read:

Rupert is pleased with himself. He feels he has made a diagnosis and organised the correct treatment. He sniggers with the medical students pointing out that the GP seems to have got it right for once, and goes on to tell them that a characteristic sufferer from gallstones has all the "F"'s: Female, Fair, Fat, Fertile and Forty. All these apply to Mrs B but she is upset to hear herself described in this fashion through the partially open door of the consulting room.

So what sort of job has Dr F done? Would Mr Spratt have made the diagnosis in his place? What happened when Mrs B first saw Dr F? In the first place, the appointment was booked not for her but for her son.

In the second place, the conversation was so disjointed that Mr Spratt would have needed a translation. The consultation at the Health Centre went like this:

Mrs B (putting down a fractious toddler) "I've been waiting nearly twenty minutes you know."

Dr F "Sorry, Mrs B, I had to go out for an emergency at the beginning of surgery and I havn't quite caught up."

Mrs B "He's no better, he needs an antibiotic."

Dr F "I don't think so, not for a cold."

Mrs B "I don't know why I bother. My period's two weeks late."

Dr F "Have you done a test?"

Mrs B "Chance would be a fine thing."

Dr F "He's still drinking then?"

Mrs B "They are always erratic. It's my hormones. I'm not putting on weight anyhow."

Dr F "Good. It would help to cut down, you know. Are you dieting?"

Mrs B "I don't eat a thing, you know, I don't know where it comes from. But I've cut out chocolate, it wasn't agreeing."

Dr F "You look like you have lost a bit. (teasing) You must be ill! "

Mrs B "Don't be like that. The indigestion has completely gone."

Dr F "When were you getting that?"

Mrs B "Now and then. Bit bad sometimes, but it's gone now."

Dr F "Did the chocolate bring it on?"

Mrs B "How did you know?"

Dr F (writing out form) "We ought to get an ultrasound, you know."

Mrs B "I'm not going up the hospital."

Dr F "Only for a test. You know, like the ones you had when you were pregnant."

Dr F has known Mrs B for ten years. She attends frequently for her children and during the consultations will discuss her husband who is verging on alcoholism. She never worries about her own health and has resisted all Dr F's attempts to help her with a diet. She is addicted to chocolate.

The SOAP analysis would have been no value. Mr Spratt would have got nowhere. In fact, he would have fallen at the first hurdle by pointing out that the consultation was for her son and not for her.

The majority of patients seen in an average general practice surgery have no serious physical illness at all. Of those that do, many will be reluctant to discuss the details with the doctor for fear of being told something they do not want to hear.

Alternatively, they may have serious psychological problems which they are embarrassed to bring up. They present repeatedly with minor, self-limiting ailments sub-consciously hoping that the GP will gently tease out the problems. A woman's main worries may, for example, relate to her loss of self-esteem since her husband lost interest in sex. Dr F's antennae will sense that something is amiss and will, possibly over a series of consultations, gently and unobtrusively probe until the problem is brought out into the open.

Rupert has heard of this sort of technique, and indeed tried it himself during the one-week compulsory GP attachment he did as a student. After he examined a middle-aged woman's thumb and found nothing, he said:

"There's nothing wrong with your thumb. How's your sex life?"

The patient told him not to be impertinent and stormed out. Rupert realised immediately that general practice was a complete waste of time. The chances of that patient discussing her real problems were put back another year.

At least thirty per cent of patients presenting to their GP with a new complaint will have underlying psychological problems. The doctor must be trained both to recognise this and to deal with it sympathetically.

Renaissance & Reformation

The mid nineteen-fifties saw a renaissance in general practice.

Despite the poor status of general practice, many outstanding and dedicated doctors had always entered it. They formed The Royal College of General Practitioners. The specialised skills that the competent family doctor needed were recognised. Guidelines for relevant postgraduate training were drawn up.

The first step was to set up a trainee year for general practice. Rather than going straight from hospital to health centre, the doctor would be attached to an experienced general practitioner, and work under his supervision, for a year. The change from hospital medicine to general practice became a supervised process rather than a traumatic event. At first it was optional. More and more elected to do the trainee year and now it is compulsory.

Next, the concept of vocational training was introduced. Rather than the doctor doing a rag bag of possibly irrelevant junior hospital jobs, a minimum hospital training period of two years is required and the jobs done must be relevant to general practice. Each job usually lasts for six months, and a typical training course might consist of appointments in:

General medicine
Paediatrics
Obstetrics & Gynaecology
Accident & Emergency

or

Paediatrics
Obstetrics & Gynaecology
Geriatrics
Orthopaedics

or

Accident & Emergency
General Medicine
ENT & Ophthalmology
Paediatrics

During the hospital jobs, the doctor on a vocational training scheme for general practice is supposed to have half a day a week off to attend the vocational training course. He will meet other trainees doing hospital jobs and discuss their relevance to general practice.

At the end of the two years hospital jobs, the doctor goes on to the one year attachment in general practice. Sometimes, and preferably, the traineeship is divided into two six-month periods either side of the hospital jobs.

Doctors may organise their own hospital jobs and trainee year. This is more flexible and gives them the opportunity to pursue their own interests. On the other hand, it means they have to apply for a new job every six months. The easier option is an organised vocational training course which many hospitals now run. Four co-ordinated hospital jobs are offered followed by a trainee year with one of the local GPs.

At the end of the training course, the would-be GP is accredited as a 'principal in general practice'.

Most GPs will take the examination for Membership of the Royal College of General Practitioners (MRCGP). It is not compulsory, nor is it likely to be. No one has yet worked out how to measure the qualities of a GP and the exam is not highly regarded.

During the hospital jobs, the GP trainee may also take one or more diploma examinations. The two commonest ones are the Diploma in Child Health (DCH) and the Diploma of the Royal College of Obstetricians and Gynaecologists (DRCOG). A reasonably well-qualified GP will have the following letters after his name:

MB BS MRCGP DCH DRCOG FPCert

However few or many letters he has, he is now entitled to apply for a position as a principal in general practice.

Becoming a GP . . .
. . . The Hard Way

The Private GP

Very few GPs are able to make a living as private practitioners with no NHS lists. They can try, but to stand any chance of success they will need considerable start-up capital, and enough savings to support themselves until they build up a list. The majority of those who succeed are in London. A few are on Harley Street and Wimpole street. Others are based in areas like Chelsea and Kensington. You will not find them in Brixton. Many of them have to supplement their earnings by acting as private doctors to the major London hotels. This is well paid but time-consuming and difficult work

Putting up a plate

A doctor may decide to start on his own as an NHS GP. As soon as he registers a patient he can claim a capitation fee of between £14.30 and £36.45 per patient, depending on the patient's age. Once he has twelve hundred patients he attracts a basic practice allowance of £6,624.[1] But however few patients he has, if he has agreed to act as their GP, he must be available twenty-four hours a day to provide medical care if and when they need it. When he starts off alone he could therefore find himself having to

[1] Full details of GP remuneration on page 59

provide a round-the-clock service for just a handful of patients.

This is the most difficult way of all to start. Few British-trained doctors do it. Single-handers who have put up their own plate are likely to be foreign, and it is hard to avoid the inference that they are only doing it because they have not been able to get any other position.

This is not to say that some single-handers are not both good and successful. Many are. But they are likely either to have broken off from a larger group practice and taken their list with them, or alternatively have applied for and been appointed to an FHSA advertised list.

The FHSA advertised list

When a single-handed GP retires, or dies in harness, there is no natural successor to the practice. The list of patients are left doctorless. The FHSA must arrange for a successor. Adverts like the one below appear in the British Medical Journal most weeks.

SURREY FHSA Applications are invited for a practice vacancy in the Surrey area due to the death of the previous practitioner six months ago. The list size is approximately 1765 patients. Surgery premises are not available and the successful doctor will be required to find his own. Applicants must be fully vocationally trained and eligible to be self employed in the United Kingdom.

Further details are available from the FHSA general manager

This stark advert gives little information about the quality of the practice; the inferences are grim. Although there is a reasonable list size, the practice will be staffed by an FHSA-appointed locum as a stop-gap. The locum obviously does not want to take the job. Many of the patients may have drifted off to other practices making the real list much lower. And there are no premises. The incoming doctor will have to find his own surgery. Although GPs receive rent re-imbursement from the FHSA, there will be no start-up capital.

There are some outstanding doctors who elect to work single-handedly. The majority of the applicants for this vacancy will be a ragbag of doctors who have either fallen out with their partners in a group practice or who have been unable to get into such a practice in the first place.

Becoming a GP . . .
. . . the easy way

Applying for a retirement or expansion vacancy in an established practice

This is the favoured way to start in general practice. Each week there are a large number of adverts in the BMJ - rarely less than twenty and sometimes two or three times as many -

from practices needing new partners.

Adverts vary from the short and to-the-point - "Doctor wanted. Please apply to..." to an expensive six paragraphs occupying a quarter-page. The only way to make a sound judgement about a practice is to visit it. Some of the most pretentious adverts are placed by some of the most incompetent GPs.

Before a doctor applies for any practice vacancy, he needs to be aware of the ways that less scrupulous partnerships may swindle him.

• Ripping off the new partner

Before the start of the NHS in 1948 a retiring GP would sell his practice to the newcomer who would then be in penury for years as he struggled to pay off the debt. NHS general practices are not allowed to sell goodwill. But they still do. They just call it "working to parity". For some reason this is allowed.

Let us suppose that James has been appointed to a group practice partnership vacancy after the retirement of Dr Crippen. His agreed terms are five years to parity. He takes over Dr Crippen's large list of three thousand patients and from day one does all the work his predecessor did. Actually, he does more, because Dr Crippen as the senior partner did not take part in the on-call rota, did not have to visit the two nursing homes, and did not do Saturday morning surgeries. James has to do all of this. Dr Crippen's share of the profits was £40,000 a year. James will start on £20,000. Each year his share will be increased by £5,000 until at the start of year five he reaches parity.

The only justification for working to parity is that all the other doctors had to do it to, and this is a way of getting back the money they lost. Two or possibly three years to parity is reasonable. Beware the practices in which it is longer.

Another wheeze that practices sometimes try and pull is to have a long 'mutual assessment period' that does not count towards parity. The new doctor is just a salaried lackey during that time and may find that at the end of the mutual assessment period, he is asked to leave.

Partnerships are supposed to be just that. Sometimes, they are autocracies, run by a despotic elderly doctor. He refuses to draw up a formal partnership agreement, refuses to let the juniors look at the books, and,most damaging of all, stops them signing on patients in their own names. If a new doctor has no formal partnership agreement and no list of his own, he has no negotiating power at all.

In summary, the following are danger signals:

➤ No partnership agreement
➤ Prolonged parity periods
➤ Prolonged mutual assessment periods separate to parity
➤ Reluctance to show the accounts
➤ A history of prospective partners only staying a few months

GPs have not the slightest interest in assessing the incoming partner's ability to practise medicine. It is assumed he is reasonably competent, but in any case it does not much matter as he will be looking after his own patients. It is important that he has had the necessary experience and qualifications to get on the various FHSA specialist lists, because these pay extra money. The most lucrative is the obstetric list, but minor operations and child surveillance are also important.

Typical adverts for practices

Let us consider four specimen adverts, and try to read between the lines.

They've got to be clearing sixty, sixty-five thousand, easy.

A business-orientated practice

Do not believe in doing their own on-call.

i.e. *public*

WESTHAMPTON A long-established forward-looking 5 partner practice with a growing list wishes to take on an additional partner to consolidate its **success** and share in an invigorating work load. We work from our own purpose built surgery and have all the usual facilities and more. Fully computerised, fundholding practice **achieving all the higher targets and Band 3 promotion**. We have an efficient well-established primary health care team. 1 in 7 rota with **extensive use of deputising service.** The incoming partner must be eligible for obstetric, minor ops and paediatric surveillance lists. **6 months mutual assessment followed by 3 years to parity**. Westhampton is a coastal town with wide range of leisure facilities, **good** schools and easy access to London and Cornwall. Applications to the practice manager.

A total three and a half years to parity is a bit on the long side but if the starting money is good and it's all in writing that may be acceptable

Summary: This advert looks tasty. If Rupert has not made it as a surgeon, he will be off to have a look.

128

Essex doctors wear Marks & Spencers blazers all the year round and in the summer add sandals and socks. They work very hard indeed and have no interest in money, which is just as well as they don't earn much: under thirty thousand. Kevin may be off here if he is a man of principle. Georgina might conceivably forsake hospital medicine and go for it is she is a God-botherer.

ESSEX Caring doctor wanted for **Christian** practice. Small lists, excellent premises. **Patients** take precedence over money and political ideology. Hand-written applications to Box 1234 BMJ.

COLCHESTER **13-26 hours** partnership available. No night duties or weekends. No daytime on call. **Interest in family planning helpful.** Full ancillary staff. Computerised appointment system. Deputising service locally. Apply to practice manager.

This practice wants a part-time female doctor. It is just that it is illegal to say so in so many words. Men need not bother to apply. They will not get a look in.

The pay will be awful: probably half a full partner's pay but three-quarters of his work load.

Rip-off merchants. Anyone mad enough to take the position will be worked very hard for as long as he can take it and paid a pittance.

Well-established group practice in Kingston requires a **salaried assistant** with a view to **partnership in 3 to 4 years.** Box 456 BMJ

Ho! Ho! Ho! Enquiries about partnership will be met with 1) excuses, and 2) an invitation to leave the practice.

Assuming the new GP can avoid the traps described above, and given average luck, he will reach parity within three years, and at about the age of thirty will have an income of around fifty thousand pounds a year. This income is guaranteed for life and whilst it may never go up a great deal, on retirement there is an index-linked pension.

It could be worse.

PRACTISING AS A GP

'Neath the Primordial Slime

The humble general practitioner was traditionally regarded as the lowest form of life in the medical profession.

The formation of the Royal College of General Practitioners and the introduction of formal and well-structured training schemes for general practice has all helped to revolutionise the standard of practice within the speciality. And it is a speciality in its own right.

The GP is on the front end of the National Health Service. When something goes wrong, it is he who is taken to task by the media. The majority of patients still have respect for the family doctor, but this respect is being eroded by the media's perception of GP incompetence, and by the GP's inability to meet the impossible demands now being made by patients.

Medical articles in the newspapers or on radio and television frequently open with, "Most GP's have not heard of... [insert name of medical condition being discussed] ...and it is advisable to see a specialist." A patient who did not see a specialist, and who became very ill, will be interviewed as 'proof' of GP incompetence. The fact that the majority of modern well-trained GPs have been treating the condition quietly and competently for years without the need for referral is not mentioned.

When medical journalists discover a condition of which they have never heard, they research it, interview a specialist who deals with it, and then write their article. Because they have never heard of it before, they assume that GPs have never heard of it either.

Take a common condition like genital herpes. It has been around since time immemorial. Genital herpes is merely one expression of a group of viruses which also cause cold sores, chicken pox and shingles. In the early '80s the tabloid press discovered herpes. Probably some journalist had an attack personally.

Genital herpes was extensively written up. It was portrayed as a new sexual plague. Doctors were flabbergasted. An attack of genital herpes, particularly the first one, can be exceedingly unpleasant but the majority of attacks are mild, and may even go unnoticed. Millions of people carry the herpes virus in their system. As a result of hysterical press exaggeration GPs were bombarded with requests for specialist referrals. Even more damaging, people with the condition were subjected to unnecessary worry and stress which, because of the press exaggeration, could not easily be dealt with by the GP.

Had HIV infections not supervened, giving the press not only the opportunity to rant about sexual excess, but also to slag off the gay community, it would probably still be topical.

The low reputation of GPs in the eyes of the media is mirrored in the attitude shown to them by hospital doctors. Most hospital doctors are patronising and dismissive of GPs. Consider the following article, which appeared in the news magazine 'Hospital Doctor'.[1]

AVALANCHE KILLS DOCTOR

A consultant paediatrician was among five doctors killed in the French Alps skiing tragedy at the weekend.

Dr Howard Fleet (43), a senior registrar at Wycombe General Hospital for 11 years, was described by colleague Dr Kim Cheetham, as 'a big man of great enthusiasm, who has a special relationship with many children and their families.'

Dr Fleet was in France on a medical education course teaching paediatrics in primary care. Four GPs were also killed.

---

[1] 'Hospital Doctor', 3rd February 1994

The Primary Health Care Team

The majority of GPs now work in partnership with one or more colleagues. The large group practices in health centres have a team of health care providers working with the doctors. Even the old-fashioned single-handed practitioner is likely to have a nurse, possibly part time, and a health visitor who has been allocated to his list.

Note that as soon as we start to describe the GP's working environment we lapse into psychobabel. No longer can we talk of the GP and the district nurse "doing their rounds". They are part of the 'primary health care team' acting in their extended role of 'health care providers'.

These terms are nonsense. They give a spurious institutional credibility to the concept of the primary health care team but in reality are only describing a system which has been in existence for over a century. Even the receptionist is part of the 'primary health care team'.

Would Dr Finlay have described Janet as a 'health care provider'?

The GP is responsible for the actions of the primary health care team but dare not regard himself as the leader. He cannot even, like the Prime Minister, claim to be *primus inter pares*. But if the practice nurse or the receptionist or the community midwife make a mistake, the GP will have to carry the can. Responsibility without control – another source of stress.

Let us look at the members of the primary health care team in more detail.

Facing *Medusa* -
The GP's Receptionist

GP receptionists often give the impression that their sole aim in life is to frustrate the reasonable needs of the patient. This is not the whole story.

They have a very difficult job and they are not well paid. They are the ham in the sandwich. They have to balance an irresistible force against an immovable object. The irresistible force is the patient. He wants to see the doctor of his choice immediately to discuss a problem that is none of the receptionist's business. He resents having to give reasons or any further information to her. He is waving a copy of the Citizens Charter. The immovable object is the doctor.

Most doctors issue standing orders to their receptionists along the following lines:

- Do not get involved in trading symptoms with the patient.

- Never give medical advice.

- Make sure that anyone with a genuine emergency is fitted in immediately.

These objectives are irreconcilable. If she declines to squeeze in a patient who turns out to have a genuine emergency the GP will be held responsible and, if the patient complains to the FHSA, may be disciplined. However busy the GP may be, he is contractually obliged to make sure he sees such patients immediately if it is necessary. It is no excuse, indeed would not even go towards mitigation, to say that it was the receptionist's fault that someone was turned away.

On the other hand, if the receptionist puts in an extra patient as an emergency with a condition that the GP regards as trivial, she will be told off.

Receptionists deal with these impossible demands by one of three strategies:

➢ They become an easy touch and always give the patients what they want. These receptionists have stressed bosses and won't last long in the job.

➢ They protect the doctor by not giving in to the patient. This makes the patient unhappy and results in an increasing number of complaints which sooner or later get the doctor into trouble.

➢ They start to act as doctors themselves. They have heard the GPs give advice to patients. It sounds easy. A bad cough? "I'll get doctor to leave a prescription out for some of those red and black capsules." Short of breath? "Why don't you take an extra water tablet. That usually helps." A temperature for two days? "Give her two spoons of Calpol [1] every four hours. That should settle her".

[1] **Calpol**: one of the most popular trademarked brands of paracetamol given to children

The third strategy is the most dangerous of all. Receptionists who adopt it are dangerous because they keep both the doctor and the patient happy.

If the doctor connives at their activity they may practise medicine in this fashion for years. The docile GP writes out the prescriptions that his receptionist suggests. Some GPs even let the receptionist have a prescription pad so that they can write the prescriptions themselves. At the end of the morning surgery, which for this sort of doctor is short and uninterrupted, they go for coffee together. As they discuss the impending marriage of her daughter, the receptionist hands the GP the bunch of prescriptions she has written out, and he signs away without checking.

It goes on. Beware the prescription that is written in one handwriting and signed in another. You may not even have that safeguard. Many prescriptions are now written by computer. They look more official but remember that the receptionist can type better than the doctor. Who really wrote the prescription?

It is a reflection of the self-limiting triviality of most illness in general practice that Category Three receptionists are rarely caught out.

So, beware! If the receptionist at your health centre always gives you what you want, she may not be giving you what you need.

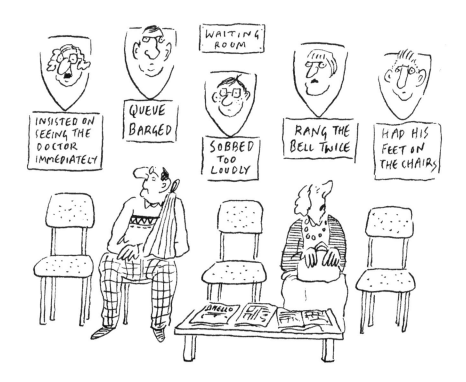

Angels in Sackcloth . . .
. . . The District Nurse

District nurses are the unsung heroes of general practice.

They are perceived as having less knowledge and status than their hospital colleagues. In reality nothing could be further from the truth. They work independently, visiting patients at home, dealing quietly and competently with serious medical conditions that their hospital colleagues would not begin to understand.

They are freed from many of the shackles imposed by their own hierarchy because senior nurses regard themselves as too important to work outside the hospital environment.

When a good nursing sister works in liaison with a competent GP the overall care provided cannot be bettered.

The Secret Service:
Health Visitors

A regular question in the examination for Membership of the Royal College of General Practitioners is:

'What is the role of the Health Visitor?'

No-one has yet written the definitive answer. Health visitors are highly paid. They are all trained nurses and many are qualified madwives as well.

They weigh babies. They visit middle class patients' houses to drink cups of tea and eat chocolate digestive biscuits.

No-one in their right mind, not even the Secretary of State for Health, would pay someone over £20,000 a year to do this. It must be a cover. But a mystifying one. Maybe they are government agents spying on the primary health care team. Speculation is rife. But still no one knows what they really do.

They are the 'secret service'.

Loony Tunes . . . the CPN

The Community Psychiatric Nurse is, as his title suggests, a trained nurse with post-qualification psychiatric experience.

At least thirty per cent of patients attending their GP with a new complaint will have underlying psychological or even psychiatric problems. These will be helped best by counselling.

The CPN provides a counselling service for patients referred by the GP. Getting such a referral depends upon the willingness of the GP to make it in the first place. Many GPs have no interest in psychological problems and so will not pick up, or will studiously ignore, all the clues a patient gives about stress and anxiety. Even if the patient is quite open about his problems and anxieties he may just be fobbed of with a prescription for Valium.

It is only the more switched-on general practices that offer a CPN counselling service, and the very fact that the offer is made means that the doctor is sympathetic and attentive to the need for such referrals.

The CPN is the torch bearer for the government's policy of community 'care'. The chronically mentally ill have been turfed out of the long-stay psychiatric wards where they had constant attention, and are now supposed to receive a weekly or fortnightly visit from the CPN. This is saving the government a lot of money. So much indeed that there is a real possibility of another CPN being appointed.

hours. He is in the invidious position of having his successes go unnoticed; only his failures are brought to light.

For every child abuse case that comes to court and thus to the attention of the tabloid press there are a thousand that have been prevented by the actions of the social work team. But let one slip through the net, and the designated social workers for the area will by hung out to dry by an unmerciless and irrational media.

When hospitals, GPs, the police, the probation service, the childrens homes and many other 'caring' agencies have a problem they cannot solve it is passed to the social worker.

It is on his desk that the buck finally stops.

The Home of Lost Causes -
Social Workers

Many practices have social workers attached to them. Social workers have the worst job of all and are cruelly lampooned.

The classic social worker is seen as a bearded, tree-hugging, earth-eating, Guardian reader, with a degree in geography or some other non-subject, who wears an anorak and muesli-coated kickers, is a member of Greenpeace, CND and Friends of the Earth, and cares deeply about "issues".

All of this is true. So what? The classic social worker is also a deeply caring and committed person. He doesn't do the job for the money, that's for sure. He works very long

The Bank Manager's Graveyard
Practice Management

Some bank managers elect to retire early, but with recent cuts and rationalisation in the banking industry, many more are being forced to go prematurely. They used to sign on the dole. Now they become GP practice managers.

Most GPs will say that they are not business men. This is not true. All GPs are business men. It is just that most of them are bad at it. Very bad.

A general practice with six partners is likely to have an ancillary staff of twenty of more. It is a business. There is a vast amount of administrative work which most doctors hate, and few do well. So most practices will appoint an administrator; a practice manager.

There is a wide variety of practice managers. Some GPs just give Mabel, the senior receptionist, a five pence pay rise and re-style her as the manager. Others advertise in the local paper and appoint an outsider. This is where the retired bank managers come in.

The large and pretentious practices advertise in the national press, offering large salaries, and appoint a young and ambitious middle-manager.

Constant Availability

"The world . . . has long ago decided that you have no working hours that anyone is bound to respect, and nothing except extreme bodily illness will excuse you in its eyes from refusing to help a man who thinks he may need your help at any hour of the day of night. Nobody will care whether you are in your bed or in your bath, on your holiday or at the theatre."

RUDYARD KIPLING (1865-1936)

"There is no harder worker in all Scotland, and none more poorly requited, than the village doctor, unless perhaps it be his horse"

SIR WALTER SCOTT (1771-1832)

The NHS GP is bound by what are called his 'terms and conditions' of service. These are laid down in 'The Red Book' which is produced by the FHSA. For the GP the above quotation from Rudyard Kipling has now been enshrined in the law. One of the terms and conditions of service is that the GP must provide medical care for his patients twenty-four hours a day, fifty-two weeks of the year. He can share this work with colleagues who are also registered GP principals with the same FHSA but if he sub-contracts any part of the work to other doctors, such as a deputising agency, he retains responsibility for their actions.

The obligation to provide twenty-four hour care is in no way mitigated by workload, personal illness, holidays, lunch or going to the lavatory. If a patient contacts a doctor with a medical problem he must be given appropriate care within a reasonable time scale. To an increasing majority of patients, now armed with a copy of the Citizens Charter,[1] appropriate means immediate. A consultant surgeon, or in reality his secretary, can always say to a patient that the clinic and operating lists are full for three months and that is a complete answer. There is no come back. If the patient dies of the condition before the operation is scheduled that is tough.

The GP has no such luxury. If he declines to see someone the same day, and that patient complains, the GP will have to defend his decision, and pressure of work is not a defence. If the patient dies from the condition, the GP will almost certainly be found to be in breach of his terms and conditions of service on a *post hoc ergo propter hoc* basis.

GPs do far fewer routine home visits than they used to, but far more so called "emergency" calls both during the working day and at night. There is a public misconception that the GP is contractually obliged to visit. This is not correct. He is only obliged to "do the right thing" and that includes a home visit if medically appropriate. The patient and the GP differ as to what they consider to be medically appropriate. If there is a dispute and a complaint follows, the FHSA complaints committee will decide. GPs end up doing visits they regard as unnecessary just to avoid such complaints.

Britain is the only country in the world where the patient has the right to summon a doctor to his bedside at any time of the day or night for any medical condition however trivial. A child vomits at midnight; a recent onset sore throat; a shift worker who cannot get to the surgery during normal working hours to have his ears syringed; an anxious university student concerned about the size of her breasts; and so on. All GPs will regale you with endless stories of such inappropriate calls.

The result of all this is stress, and more stress, for the doctor. The BMA has been pressurising the Government into making changes and as this book is being written it looks like something will happen. The government has decided that doctors will no longer be obliged to visit patients out-of-hours. This is not a concession. They never were *obliged* to visit. All that will happen now is that the doctor-patient interface will be more fraught as the patient tries to persuade or bully the doctor into visiting. And the doctor is still in difficulties because if it is decided retrospectively that he should have visited, he will be reprimanded.

Turn the page for a guide to the complaints procedure.

---

[1] The Citizens Charter does not specifically apply to GPs. Try telling the punter that.

Complaining about a GP

GPs are uniquely placed in triple jeopardy. Any complaint that is made against them can be taken to three different bodies, and to all simultaneously if the complainant wishes.These bodies are:

1. The Law Courts
2. The General Medical Council (GMC)
3. The FHSA

GPs can be sued in the law courts for negligence just like anyone else. A few are. This is not a serious threat for the GP because it happens rarely. Similarly, complaints to the GMC, other than vexatious nonsense which is thrown out immediately, are also rare. Both the courts and the GMC exercise their powers in a defined judicial fashion; the doctor can be legally represented; the decisions taken are fair and predictable. A doctor who has been grossly negligent and harmed or even killed a patient can hardly complain that the action taken was "unfair".

The problem for the GP is the FHSA complaints procedure. The GP is bound by his terms and conditions of service, and any complaint made by a patient will be interpreted in the light of those terms and conditions.

The system works as follows. The FHSA receives a letter of complaint. This goes to someone who has a grand title like The Patient Services Facilitator but who is in fact just a typist. A copy of the letter is sent to the doctor asking for his comments. His comments are then sent to the complainant who decides if the answer satisfies the complaint.

If he wishes to continue with the complaint most FHSAs will offer him an informal arbitration scheme dealt with by a lay member of the FHSA. The complainant must consent to the informal process. If he does the matter can be settled by negotiation.

If he wishes to continue with the formal complaint the papers are sent to the Chairman of the Medical Services Committee, which is the FHSA Committee whose sole purpose is to deal with complaints. The Chairman will decide from the papers whether there is sufficient evidence to justify a formal hearing in front of the full committee. His decision is only a recommendation and is not communicated to either party until it has been accepted by the next full meeting of the FHSA.

If the decision is that there are *not* sufficient grounds for a hearing the complainant may appeal to the Secretary of State.

If there *is* to be a hearing, a date will be set and the parties informed. The hearing is in front of the full Medical Services Committee which has both medical and lay people on it. Neither party may be represented by a lawyer, but each may bring someone to speak on their behalf. Both sides may call witnesses and may put questions to the opponent's witnesses. Each is given an opportunity to sum up and then the committee retires to make its decision. The decision is only a recommendation and has to be accepted by the FHSA at its next meeting.

If the decision goes against the doctor he is formally found to have been "in breach of his terms and conditions of service." He will most likely be reprimanded and warned to adhere more closely to them in the future. Such a reprimand is a stain on a doctor's professional reputation and is dreaded. In exceptional cases the FHSA can fine him by withholding part of his remuneration.

But the complainant is also unhappy. To him, a reprimand is nothing. He wants blood. He thinks the doctor has "got off".

Both the complainant and the doctor may appeal to the Secretary of State, and the truly determined could go beyond that and get judicial review.

It may sound reasonable and judicial, but it is not. Both the complainant and the doctor are usually dissatisfied with the process. There is incredible administrative delay – sometimes over a year and longer if there are appeals to the Secretary of State. FHSAs pay mediocre salaries and so get mediocre staff who have no insight into the stress suffered by the doctor or the anger felt by the patient.

There is nothing worse than a barrack-room lawyer let loose in a quasi-judicial hearing. The MSC service committee hearings are kangaroo courts. They make trained lawyers despair. The onus of proof is reversed. However vexatious and unfounded the complaint may be, the doctor will have to prove his innocence rather than the patient prove guilt. The committee has not a clue about rules of evidence and listens to any amount of hearsay and unsubstantiated gossip. The lay members of the committee are local worthies and do-gooders who do not have a real job but do have a political agenda to "get a fair deal for the patient". The doctors on the MSC are a precious lot who enjoy committee work. Who is looking after their patients during the hearing, one wonders?

Complainants do not understand that the hearing is about "terms and conditions of service" as laid down in the red book. These are esoteric, specific and not all-encompassing. A doctor could keep within the terms of service and still be grossly negligent. Conversely, being found to be in breach of them does not necessarily provide any evidence of negligence that a court would entertain.

Last year, a GP who was facing a service committee hearing for a relatively minor complaint committed suicide.

The Seventy-Nine Per Centers

In a national opinion poll of GPs carried out in early 1994, 79 per cent of GPs polled said they would like to give the job up. Why is this?

The strain of having to be constantly available, coupled with the ever present and increasing possibility of an FHSA service committee hearing, has had a profoundly destructive effect. GPs are at breaking point. They went into the profession with the naive idea that they would be family doctors. Of course they expected to provide an emergency service for serious illness; by serious illness they meant strokes, heart attacks, acute asthma, appendicitis and so on. They had no inkling of the public's readiness to call them out for trivial ailments, nor of the abuse they would be subjected to if they demurred or declined to provide an immediate home consultation.

The service is free, so it is abused.

Some say GPs are idle, overpaid and inefficient; that they should stop whingeing and get on with the job.

Maybe.

But there are approximately twenty-eight thousand GPs practising in England and Wales. They cannot all be like that. Most of them are ordinary, decent men and women who went into a caring profession with high and honourable ambitions. Why do over seventeen thousand of them want to give up?

The demands of constant availability mean that many GPs have come to regard the patient as "the enemy". When the surgery opens in the morning, there is a "repel boarders" feeling.

An eminent Home Counties GP, who is one of the senior partners in a large and successful practice and the postgraduate tutor at a district general hospital, recently said the following:

"We monitor our out-of-hours calls very carefully. If any patients use the service too much we throw them off our list. Recently, we found we were getting a lot of calls from one particular street in a council estate in our area, so we removed

the whole street.

It is important that it is not made too easy for the patient to get hold of the doctor. Whenever I get a night call, I always insist that the patient meets me at the surgery. That is much more time consuming for me, but it teaches the patient a lesson. I always try to assess the socio-economic group of the patient who calls me in the evenings and at weekends. I work out which is likely to be their favourite television programme. Then I tell them to meet me at the surgery in the middle of Neighbours or Panorama as appropriate. These people have got to learn."

All GPs understand the emotion running through this ststement. But what would the patient think? Is it important that "it is not made too easy for the patient to get hold of his doctor"? What happens if the Fire Brigade takes the same view? This was one GP's strategy for avoiding the stress of being on-call. He is not alone.

GPs have ex-directory telephone numbers. Most of them choose to live outside their practice area. When they are not on-call they make sure they are so *incommunicado* that members of their staff, or even their families, are unable to find them. They adopt all sorts of odd strategies to avoid patients during their free time.

Some GPs leave their phone off the hook. It is amazing how long they get away with it. Strangely, if people cannot get through to the doctor at all, they seem to accept it and wait until the next day. By then the medical 'emergency' has got better spontaneously and they have forgotten about it. The GPs who get the complaints are the ones who answer the phone and then argue about the merits of a visit.

Other GPs hand over all their on-call to a deputising service. These provide an out-of-hours service of variable quality, and a large percentage of GPs are not prepared to use them.

There is a glimmer of light on the horizon for GPs in the form of co-operatives. Co-operatives are non-profit-making organisations owned and run by GPs. They were founded in Lancashire over ten years ago. They have been developed in Kent and most recently a large co-operative called **Thamesdoc** was started in the North Surrey and Kingston area. **Thamesdoc** now has over one hundred and fifty GP members and is providing out-of-hours cover for about a quarter of the population of Surrey, and most of the Kingston and Richmond area.

GPs in co-operatives still do all their own on-call, without the use of deputies or locums, but they work in six-hour shifts rather than all night or all weekend, and have a car and a driver. Both patients and GPs find the system excellent. The only problem is that the GPs have to fund the service out of their own pockets. It is costing each member of **Thamesdoc** four thousand to five thousand pounds a year to provide the service.

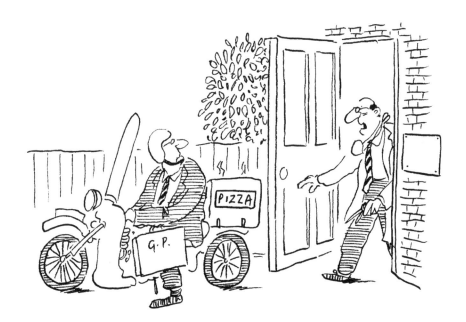

"Dammit Roger – it's only *medical* emergencies we have to answer."

NURSES AND MADWIVES

Doctors' Handmaidens
THE NURSES

The nursing profession has come a long way since the days of Florence Nightingale. Modern nurses do not see themselves as the doctor's assistant, and most certainly not as his handmaiden.

Entrance requirements for nursing have become stiffer and stiffer. It is now possible to do a university degree in nursing. The teenage girl wishing to train at a London teaching hospital will find that there are similar A-level requirements as for university. So why bother to do nursing? A good question.

Girls who would make excellent nurses are kept out by the academic requirements. Those who can meet the requirements would be better off going to university. Many of them come to regard traditional nursing tasks as beneath their dignity.

ing bottoms and preventing bedsores. Some of the old style nurses still do this.

The modern teaching hospital nurse, with her A-levels and her university degree, is far too clever to carry out these mundane and unpleasant tasks. They are delegated to the 'ancillary' staff. Ancillary nurses, who are not nurses at all, now do the nursing. The nurse who should be doing the nursing sits at the nursing station pretending to be a doctor.

The ancillary staff do not have any formal medical training, and make mistakes. Diabetic patients are given high sugar meals; patients who should be starved before surgery are fed; elderly immobile patients who should be turned in bed are left unturned and develop bedsores.

The nurses, meanwhile, are sitting at their consoles pretending to read ECGs and to interpret complex biochemical investigations. They do not take responsibility for these 'interpretations' but drive the doctors mad with their helpful suggestions.

Bums and Bedsores

The layman might assume that a nurse's main professional role is . . . well, nursing; looking after the patient, dealing with bedpans, powder-

Doctors cure, nurses care

The nursing hierarchy has long been trying to demonstrate that the nursing profession is as important as the medical profession. No-one ever thought it was not, until the senior nurses gave vent to their paranoia. In an attempt to increase the status of nurses they have shrouded the profession in a complex hierarchy of rules and regulations which has succeeded only in robbing nurses of the power of thought. They are discouraged from exercising initiative and subjected to horrific disciplinary sanctions if they are seen to step out of line. This leads to frustrations, which they take out on the houseman.

Senior nurses resent the superior status of junior doctors. When a new housman arrives on the ward his knowledge of practical medicine is zero. Worse than that, really, because he is under the illusion that his recent success in medical finals means something. He is easy meat. Nurses break a new houseman in every six months. They lack theoretical knowledge but floor him with questions about practical management.

Snakes and Ladders

In the children's game you climb the ladders and slide down the snakes. In the nursing hierarchy game, you climb the ladders and get bitten by the snakes.

The great and the good of the nursing profession are a peculiar lot. They are hell bent on destroying their own professional standing and autonomy.

The career structure makes patient contact and promotion incompatible. The competent nurse will rise to the level of Ward Sister in her late twenties. If she wants further prefer-

ment she has to go into administration. Many nurses went into the profession because they enjoyed looking after the patients. They do not want to be administrators. And so, either they stay as Ward Sisters at the top of their grade but with no further prospects of career advancement, or they take a sideways step into midwifery. They may even decide to join the secret service, and train as health visitors.

Many are married, and in their late twenties or early thirties decide to have children. The nursing profession is largely female. You would expect it, of all professions, to make comprehensive and sympathetic provision for maternity leave. If an experienced nurse wants to return to her profession, a refresher course lasting a few weeks, followed by an attachment to a colleague working at her level of experience, would enable her to return to her previous job.

There are no such provisions. She is not welcomed back. The system is such that she is actually discouraged. If she comes back, she will lose much of her seniority.

A thirty-five year old who has been an experienced Ward Sister on a busy medical ward will be faced with the prospects of returning to be bossed around by a newly-qualified twenty-two year old Staff Nurse.

Many nurses never return. Their training goes to waste. If they do any nursing at all, it is probably just the odd session in a private nursing home. The cream of the profession is lost.

So who stays in nursing and climbs the career ladder? The oddballs. A high proportion of the senior nurses are unmarried. They are happier to work in administration because they never enjoyed patient contact in the first place. They are not good with patients; they are not good with people. Nor are they any good as administrators. Why should they be? They were never trained for it.

How does this odd group of women pass its time? Like all administrators, good or bad, they issue rules and regulations, directives and policy documents, job descriptions and protocols; a never-ending stream of bureaucratic psychobabel which is destroying a once proud profession. They have not done any hands-on nursing for years, and when they did do it most of them were hopeless at it. But they still see themselves as nurses and feel it is important to issue guidelines on clinical management.

Toeing the line

Most trades unions and professional organisations aim to protect the interests of their members. It is hard to understand how the Royal College of Nursing (RCN) can claim to be doing that.

It sees its role more as policing the profession. The disciplinary code it has for nurses who step out of line is harsh. Nurses are frightened of it. Their perpetual cry now when asked to perform a duty that they have been doing for years is "No, we are not covered to do that."

The nursing hierarchy has lost sight of, or never understood, the

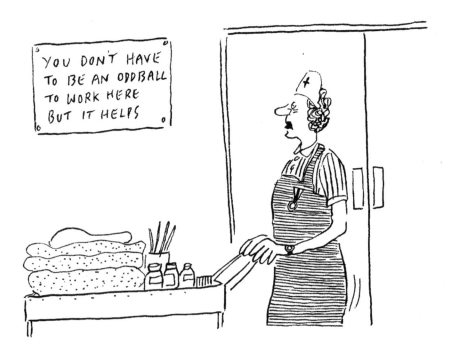

general legal principals governing professional negligence. The legal standard for judging whether a professional is at fault is clear cut. He is required to exercise the skill of a reasonably competent practitioner in his field. No more; no less. He will not be adjudged to have failed to come up to the required standard if a respectable body of opinion within that profession - and not necessarily the majority opinion - would find his actions acceptable.

Applying this sort of standard, there *is* scope for initiative, for judgement, and most of all for original thought. But the RCN is frightened of independent judgement and strangles any attempts made by nurses to act autonomously.

Male Nurses

One of the salvations of the nursing profession has been its acceptance of male nurses, characteristically reluctant and tardy though it was. The spinster hierarchy fought long and hard against the idea of equal opportunities for men within the profession, but lost.

Male nurses are still given a bad time during their training by the old-fashioned sisters, and particularly by the administrative hierarchy.

It is not true to say that all male nurses are gay. Many of them are, though. Just as an enormous number of gay men are artistic and creative, they seem also to have a special talent for patient care.

Madwives

Madwives are specialised nurses. On a percentage basis, they have in their midst the largest collection of oddballs and eccentrics in the whole nursing profession. Indeed, they are the most unusual group of people in the NHS; more unusual even than the psychiatrists. Their role in childbirth is controversial and jealously guarded.

Many madwives are unmarried and have not had children themselves. They have a subconscious desire to punish women who do have babies. As a result of their attitude, pregnant women are led to believe that childbirth is a competition, and that the only winner is the one who gets through labour:

1. without pain relief
2. without forceps
3. without an episiotmy [1]
4. without stitches
5. without whingeing

Women who cannot meet these criteria are made to feel like failures.

Ten Green Bottles or an O.B.E.

Madwives can be divided into two categories; the old and the new.

[1] A surgical procedure whereby a small neat cut is made in the vagina to prevent a large ragged tear

146

The Old-Fashioned Madwife . . .

➤ Is a spinster.

➤ Regards childbirth as a necessary but unpleasant and messy business.

➤ Knows that it is not painful and gets angry with the tiresome and weak-minded women who scream in labour.

➤ Regards pubic hair as tainted, and the vulva and perineum as a "dirty" area. A shave and a bath are essential before a baby passes through.

➤ Is appalled by a woman's tendency to open her bowels during labour. This filthy and disgusting habit can be avoided by a large dose of castor oil and an enema on admission to the ward.

➤ Is not amused that her antenatal ritual is known as the Oil, Bath & Enema.

➤ Will reluctantly let a women have a pethidine injection but then tell her that it is her own fault that it made her vomit.

➤ Whisks the new born baby away to perform unnecessary madwifery rituals without letting mother have a cuddle.

➤ Worships the consultant.

➤ Is called Doris.

The New Age Madwife . . .

➤ Is married to a social worker.

➤ Has three children called Flora, Harry and Daisy.

➤ Encourages the husband to get into bed with his wife during labour.

➤ Is at her happiest joining the naked husband and wife in the birthing pool.

➤ Thinks that singing Ten Green Bottles is a better painkiller than an epidural.

➤ Thinks that blood, meconium, urine, liquor, and faeces have mystical healing powers.

➤ Insists that the mother has a long cuddle with the new born baby even if it is not breathing properly and the paediatrician is desperate to resuscitate it.

➤ Encourages mother and father to eat the placenta.

➤ Does not believe in doctors.

➤ Is called Beth.

Neither Doris nor Beth exist. They are extremes. All madwives are composites of both, but with a definite tendency in one or other direction.

Patronising the Punter

"The ultimate indignity is to be given a bedpan by a stranger who calls you by your first name."

MAGGIE KUHN (1905 -)
The Observer 1978

Madwives feel they have the right to use a patient's first name without invitation. The woman attending the ante-natal clinic will be referred to, politely and courteously, as Mrs Jones, or by the politically conscious as Ms Jones. Such good manners disappear in the labour ward. A women in labour is in pain and is disadvantaged. The madwife calls her "Julie". She will not ask if she wants to be addressed by her first name. Such familiarity may be acceptable if it is a community madwife who has seen the patient all through her pregnancy and knows her well. It is not acceptable from a stranger. Especially as there is no question of it being a reciprocal transaction. It goes, "Hello Julie, I'm Sister Smith."

The madwife would maintain that she is only being friendly and the informality puts patients at ease. Maybe. Sometimes. More often it is the madwife exercising power over a patient at a disadvantage. Doctors do not use patients' first names.

Politicising the Vagina

Madwives worship the vagina. Their main objective during childbirth is to protect vaginal integrity and in particular to avoid an episiotomy. They write the words "Intact perineum" in the patient's notes as though it is a political triumph.

This shows a remarkable lack of knowledge of human anatomy, and no understanding of other purposes for which women like to use their vaginas.

At the most difficult and painful part of a delivery, when the baby's

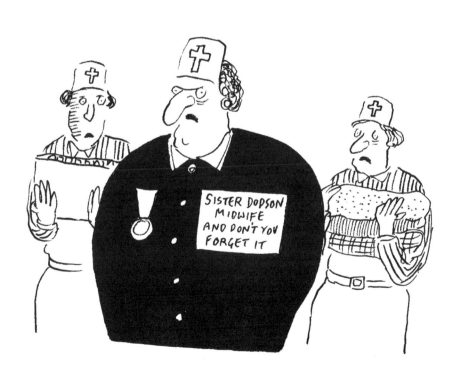

head is being born, the vagina may suddenly tear. Tears may be small, but can be large and multiple, sometimes catastrophically extending into the rectum. A tear going into the rectum, a third degree tear, needs careful surgical repair to avoid faecal incontinence, and even in the best hands, the results may not be perfect.

Even when there is no tear, and the madwife can write her magic words "intact perineum", there may be underlying damage. The vagina is a forgiving organ. But it has to stretch enormously during childbirth. There are large numbers of elderly women, who had their children in a less enlightened age, who suffer from constant urinary leakage and faecal incontinence. A major cause of these problems is damage done during childbirth. Much of that damage can be avoided.

Suturing vaginal tears is an important surgical procedure. Unfortunately, it is usually done by medical students at the beginning of their training or, even worse, by madwives who have had no surgical training at all. The medical student at least has some knowledge of anatomy.

Suturing vaginas in a rite of passage for medical students. Medical machismo demands that however difficult the repair, the registrar should not be disturbed. Such repairs are often done badly. The madwife is even more reluctant to ask the doctor for help because in matters of childbirth she regards herself as an oracle.

A small and timely episiotomy will facilitate the easier delivery of the baby; it leaves a cut that is easily visualised and can thus be completely repaired. It will protect the women from lifelong perineal problems.

No-one argues that all women should have an episiotomy, nor that none should have one. The decision should be taken, though, on clinical not political grounds. Madwives who delight in the superficially intact, but stretched and bruised, perineum should be made to work for six months in a urology clinic dealing with incontinent middle-aged and elderly women.

The Great Escape

Having escaped the trauma of the labour ward, the new mother and baby now has to survive a different form of madwife on the post-natal ward. To minimise the damage, the wise mother plans to escape as soon as possible.

The post-natal madwife's mission in life is:

1. To destroy the mother's confidence by mystifying the basics of caring for new born babies.

2. To dry up the mother's breast milk.

3. To connive with commercial companies to poison the babies

4. To keep the mother in hospital as long as possible.

Mystical Rituals

#1: Topping and Tailing

"Have you learnt to 'top and tail' yet?" will be the anxious question whispered round the maternity ward. This mysterious process is built up to the status of a goat-shaggers' initiation ceremony. The madwife will not

NURSES AND MADWIVES   149

let a mother go home until she can do it.

'Topping and tailing' means changing the dirty nappy, powdering the bum and sloshing a bit of water on the baby's head.

#2: Rooming

Should the baby be roomed in at the mother's bedside or taken to the nursery?

Madwives have a variety of theories, all perfectly plausible, and all contradictory. The babies get bounced backwards and forwards as the shifts of madwives come and go.

The answer is that it does not much matter whether the baby is roomed in with its mother or put in the nursery. The mother should be allowed to decide.

Breast milk

There is no moral or medical absolute that says that new mothers must breast-feed. Feeding babies is a question of fashion. There are advantages to both breast and bottle and although most doctors would say that breast-feeding for at least the first three months is the best policy, the decision should be made by the mother.

Madwives do not believe in choice. They tell mothers that they must breast-feed. They may well have a special breast-feeding room. There will be no bottle-feeding room so the bottle-feeders feel like second class citizens.

Years ago the fashionable belief was that new born babies should be

starved for the first twenty-four hours. This is wrong. It is important that they feed. But the need for feeding has become an obsession for madwives. Ironically, their approval of breast-feeding is only a pretence. The truth is, they are frightened of it. Breasts are not transparent and do not have lines on them to show the number of ounces of milk they contain. Bottles do. Madwives are not at peace until they can measure a baby's milk intake. That means bottle-feeding. To achieve this objective, they adopt strategies, maybe unconsciously, to put mothers off breast-feeding.

They stick babies on breasts at the wrong time when the mother is uncomfortable. They start criticising the mother for not having enough milk and insist on topping up the baby with bottle milk thus making their original accusation a self-fulfilling prophecy. They then 'tut tut', saying "What a shame you failed at breast-feeding" and produce a bottle of formula. At a stroke they have achieved two of their objectives; they have destroyed the mother's confidence and got the baby on the bottle.

Poisoning babies

There is a conspiracy between madwives and commercial companies to get sugar into babies as soon as possible so that they develop a sweet tooth and start rejecting food that does not have added sugar. The madwives prepare the ground by drying up the breast milk.

Commercial companies supply post-natal wards with gift packs containing high sugar rusks, cereals and baby food. Everyone likes a freebie. None of these is necessary for the baby, who will survive quite happily, and indeed is nutritionally better off, on breast milk or formula. But still the madwives dole out the packs.

Why?

unwise not to comply. But if the doctors are happy for you to go, and you want to go, you should. Don't let the madwife bully you into signing a form saying you have discharged yourself against medical advice. You have not.

False imprisonment

Most ante-natal clinics suggest to mothers that they book for a short, medium or long stay in the post-natal ward. First time mothers are encouraged to have a long stay.

Having booked for a particular length of stay, madwives like mothers to stick to the arrangement. If they have booked a three-day stay and ask to go on the second day the madwife's eyebrows furrow, her brain circuitry begins to overheat, and she spouts out a whole load of bogus reasons as to why the mother should stay. "But you haven't learnt to top and tail yet" or "Your breast milk is not established" or, and this is the classic, "The community madwife hasn't been informed."

This is complete nonsense. Having a baby is not a criminal offence. You are not in custody. You are free to leave when you wish and it is not for the madwife to stop you. The hospital madwife likes to inform the community madwife before you escape. This is because the community madwife has a statutory duty to visit you at home to finish off drying up the breast milk if the job was not done in hospital.

Of course, no prudent patient leaves against medical advice. If the obstetrician or paediatrician advises staying a little longer, it would be

The GP as Gatekeeper

Entry into the British health care system, apart from emergencies taken straight to Casualty departments, is through the GP.

Over ninety percent of all doctor-patient contacts are dealt with at this level. Lapsing into psychobabel, this is the 'primary health care system.' The patient is not deemed clever enough to be able to refer himself to hospital – the 'secondary health care system.' There is also a tertiary health care system – the super-specialist hospitals, such as the Royal Hospital for Sick Children at Great Ormond Street. (GOS) The Consultants there have decided that GPs are not clever enough to refer patients directly to them. Patients must first go to an 'ordinary' paediatrician at an 'ordinary' hospital. If the medical condition is rare enough or interesting enough it will then be accepted. There is an exception to this rule: GPs are clever enough to refer *private* patients to G.O.S. consultants.

The GP thus acts as the gatekeeper to the National Health Service. The average GP has around two thousand patients and the average patient consults his doctor three and a half times a year. The average GP therefore sees about twenty-five patients a day.

Ten per cent of primary health care contacts will generate a secondary health care referral. Individual GP referral rates vary enormously from as low as five percent to as high as thirty.

• The GPs with low referral rates say that their experience and clinical acumen enables them to deal with many problems that their less experienced colleagues would refer.

• The GPs with high referral rates say that their low-referring colleagues have such atrophied clinical abilities that they do not diagnose the conditions that need referral in the first place.

In spite of frequent harangues in the media about poorly-educated GPs the objective evidence is that the system works well, and that the standard of primary health care delivery in the UK is unmatched throughout the world.

For better or worse, the system is here to stay. For one reason only. Whether or not it is the best system in the world, it is one of the cheapest. The British GP provides ninety per cent of the health care in the country for ten per cent of the total health care budget. A good buy for any government

---

Before Margaret

The Profligate GP

Perhaps because the primary health care service has always been so cheap to run, there have never been any proactive cost restraints on GP referrals. In the past, individual doctor's referral costs were rarely monitored and when they were the information was not fed back to the doctor so that he could modify and improve his behaviour. The family doctor could be as idle and as out-of-date as he wished. If he chose to clog up the local dermatologist's clinic with veruccas rather than treat them himself, he could. GPs have always exercised an unfettered right to refer and prescribe without regard to cost.

Bearing in mind that to treat veruccas himself a GP has to buy all the necessary equipment, kit out a treatment room and pay for the nurse's time, all out of his own pocket, who could blame him for referring the patient to hospital?

Hospital Incompetence

Hospitals have their own problems.

The perceived moral absolute of health care for all, free at the point of entry, as provided by the NHS, bred all the usual inefficiencies seen in nationalised industries:

> ➤ Diffused and inefficient leadership. The buck is never passed; the buck never stops; the buck has not been **invented** in the NHS hospital.

> ➤ No financial or career incentive for administrators to improve.

> ➤ Gross over-manning with an over-priced and inefficient ancillary workforce. When Guy's Hospital became a Trust, one of the first things it did was make three hundred porters redundant.

The worst abuse has been the explosion in the numbers of administrators. It has been much studied, but never explained. The *ODPH* can now provide that explanation. Administrative growth works on The Coat Hanger Principle.

The Coat Hanger Principle

1. Go into the spare bedroom in your house.

2. Open the empty wardrobe.

3. Put two wire frame coat hangers in the wardrobe and lock the doors.

4. Close the bedroom door and go away.

5. Return in six months. Open the wardrobe. There are fifty-eight wire coat hangers in it.

And so it is in the NHS hospitals. Nobody knows where the administrators come from. When a new administrator arrives, he immediately takes the following actions:

- Appoints three assistants.
- Buys himself and his assistants lap top computers.
- Refurnishes the offices.
- Reserves himself a space in the hospital car park.
- Issues a mission statement.
- Ask a random sample of twenty-five per cent of the medical staff to provide a ten-thousand-word document describing their clinical work activities. This to be done in their spare time.
- Holds a committee meeting.
- Sacks twenty-five per cent of the doctors on the grounds that their work activity studies show them to be superfluous to requirements.

Grafted on top of all this administrative inefficiency was budgetary incompetence of a high order. The level of NHS funding is notionally based on need but in fact is last year's fund plus an agreed additional percentage which bears some relationship to current inflation rates but is basically the lowest amount of money that the Government can get away with politically. Governments never fund for a future when they may not be in office.

Once a hospital has received its annual budget, the various departments fight it out for as large a slice of the cake as they can get. Glamorous and politically powerful departments like cardiac surgery in London teaching hospitals get far more than psycho-geriatrics in Salford.

Any health service, however structured, is a bottomless pit of expenditure and could consume the whole Gross National Product if allowed. The problem is universal. It is common to hear Americans criticising the "socialised medicine" of the NHS; they will in particular mention the waiting lists. Waiting lists are a method of rationing health care and controlling expenditure. They are at least fair in their impact. The Americans limit health care in a different way. They exclude thirty million of their citizens from it altogether. In the USA, health care is not free at the point of entry. Those thirty million cannot afford even to join a waiting list. They are the poor, the disadvantaged, the inner-city slum dwellers. They are often black or Puerto Rican. They are no-one's constituents.

In the UK over the last seven years there has been a radical, root and branch change in the mode of health care delivery. The reason for, and the impetus behind, this change can best be summarised in three words: Margaret Hilda Thatcher.

After Margaret

Margaret Hilda Thatcher believed passionately in the efficiency of a free market economy and in the merits of privatisation. The NHS was not to be exempt. If market forces could be introduced into health care, she was convinced they would automatically bring higher standards of care and cost-efficiency.

The new buzz words would be "purchasers" and "providers" – fundholding GPs and trust-status hospitals all competing in a free market place.

The purchase of health care could have been entrusted to the patient.

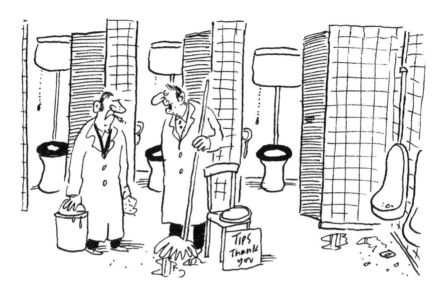

"The managers say we've just got to put more bums on seats."

They could have been allowed continued free access to the NHS with the bill for each contact being sent to the government. Such a system exists in parts of Canada. But in England it would have caused an immediate and exponential increase in health care costs.

To maintain control it was decided to appoint purchasers to act upon behalf of the patients. The purchasers were to be the GPs. They would be known as fundholders. Provided they met certain criteria about size of practice and could demonstrate a degree of administrative efficiency they would negotiate and receive a budget from the Regional Health Authority and would then be allowed to spend it as they saw fit on purchasing health care for their patients. They could spend the money in the NHS or in the private sector at their discretion. What is more, if at the end of the year they came in under budget, they could spend those savings on their own practices.

GPs with small lists, or those who did not wish to fundhold, would rely on the District Health Authority to place block contracts with local hospitals on their behalf. This would free them from administrative work, but severely limit their choice of referral hospitals.

The *Advantages* of the System

From any political view point the new system has many advantages and has without doubt improved hospital efficiency. In particular:

➢ The GP is an educated consumer of health care and is better able to monitor the quality of care received by a patient than the patient himself.

➤ Trust status hospitals are prevented from pursuing profit in the way some American hospitals do. GP purchasers will not allow the patients to be over-investigated nor will the syndrome of 'two operations are better than one' prevail.

➤ Patients are "ring-fenced". If someone is admitted, for example, for a hernia repair, inter-disciplinary referrals to sort out co-existing minor problems that are already being treated by the GP will not be funded. The dermatologist will not get paid for going to see the hernia patient's verucca, and so he does not go.

➤ The money follows the patient. Efficient hospitals attract more revenue and thrive whilst inefficient hospitals "wither on the vine". Resources become concentrated where they are best used.

The *Disadvantages* of the System

➤ Fundholding has introduced another tier of inequality into the NHS. Patients of fundholding practices receive better and faster care than those of non-fundholding practices. The government denies this. They say that trust hospitals are not allowed to "fast-track" fundholding patients. This is political duplicity of the highest order. The whole purpose of the new system is for purchasers to negotiate improved care for their patients. There is no other reason for doing it.

➤ It has created an unhealthy and antagonistic relationship between GPs and hospital doctors. The fundholder's budget has not been conjured up out of thin air. It has been taken, pound for pound, from the hospital's budget. If the local hospital does not attract all the local GP fundholder patients, it will be in financial difficulties. The logic of the system breaks down. Hospitals have immutable, fixed costs, however many patients they treat, and will have difficulty meeting those costs if, say, ten per cent of their budget, the difference between profit and loss, is removed. The hospital doctors have therefore to court the GPs they once ignored, and they resent it.

➤ Whatever Margaret Hilda may think, the laws of supply and demand do not apply to health care. There is finite supply and infinite demand, and, given that the health service remains free at the point of entry, there is no real price mechanism to control the relationship between the two. Purchasers and providers are playing with monopoly money.

➤ An enormous administrative burden has fallen onto the GPs. Although fundholding practices are paid a management allowance to take on extra staff, the GPs themselves are not paid for the extra administrative work. Many are putting in an extra ten to twenty hours a week. Morale is low.

➤ In business, projects that are uneconomic are scrapped. In health care, patients may well be beyond economic repair but they are not scrapped. They are referred to geriatricians for less intensive but still expensive care.

In conclusion, as an economic model the health care market is fundamentally flawed. It was, for example, realised immediately that long term psychiatric and geriatric care could not be a source of profit, and so those areas were excluded. Intensive medical care is expensive; a GP fundholder who had to pay for heart surgery or renal dialysis could spend his whole budget on three patients. Further exclusions and expenditure stop losses were introduced.

In order to ensure that the new system survived, the Thatcher government ended up doing everything it purported to detest; it meddled with and sought to control the internal "free market" health economy.

The Future:
Political Ping Pong

The future of the new system depends entirely on the result of the next election. An incoming Labour government is pledged to make root and branch changes; in particular it is likely to stop hospitals giving priority to patients from fundholding practices. No-one, apart from Tory health ministers, denies that it goes on. But if it is stopped, many GPs will see little purpose in continuing as fundholders.

The greatest concern is that a future administration might emasculate the internal health market, destroy all the benefits it has introduced, and leave behind only the paperwork. It is easier to create a bureaucracy than to destroy it.

HOW TO CHOOSE A DOCTOR

Choosing a GP

"When I go, ten per cent of my patients will, on balance, be sad. Ten per cent of them will, on balance, be glad. Eighty per cent will not notice."

HOME COUNTIES GP

On retiring after 40 years in practice

If you live in the same area as your parents you probably carry on with the same GP who has looked after the family for years. He has been handed down by your parents and is almost a family retainer. With a bit of luck, he is a trusted family friend as well. Or that is how you like to see him.

But if you move to a new area you have to go through the process of selecting a GP yourself. How do you do it? Does it matter? Most people do it on a geographical basis; they sign on with the practice that is nearest to their house. Such random selection is all well and good for mobile young professionals in their late twenties who have no children and only go to the doctor for contraceptive advice and immunisations before their exotic holidays. As they get older and have children, and even older and start to become ill, it does matter.

Single-hander or group practice?

Personal service is important. Patients like to see 'their' doctor rather than one of the partners. But this is not the most important criterion. Countless surveys have shown that the main thing patients want is doctor availability; and that his availability is more important than his identity.

If this applies to you, you should always join a group practice. There will be howls of anguish from the single-handed GPs, some of whom are outstanding. Tough. The fact is that when they take holidays, when they have a half-day, when they have a weekend off, their patients' care is delegated either to a deputising service or to another doctor in the area who shares an on-call rota. Either way, the deputy will not have access to your notes and will not be able to provide anything like as efficient a service.

If a single-hander is always available, in other words takes no time off, he is mad or bad or both and sooner rather than later will burn out.

How to assess a practice

Go and sit in the waiting room with a copy of the *ODPH* and watch and listen. What kind of receptionists are there? Are they polite? Are they obviously trying to repel boarders? Worst of all, are they trying to act as doctors themselves by advising over the counter about medical conditions?

All GPs should have a practice brochure. Read it. If there is not one, take your business elsewhere. Are the surgery times offered reasonable? Is there a female doctor? Do they have clinics for specific conditions such as diabetes and asthma? Are the arrangements for out-of-hours emergencies clearly displayed in the brochure?

Having decided that the practice looks like the right one for you, tell the receptionist that you are thinking of joining and would like an appointment with one of the partners to discuss the services offered. Some practices will not allow this. Ask why not and then take your business elsewhere.

Fundholder or non-fundholder?

Fundholding is covered in more detail in Chapter Ten on page 151, but patients should be under no illusion that the fundholding system has introduced yet another tier of inequality into the NHS. Patients of fundholding

practices get much swifter and more efficient care from the NHS. The politicians deny it; the hospitals pretend they do not do it; the GPs are embarrassed by it. Morally it stinks but it is a fact of life.

Always join a fundholding practice if you have the opportunity.

Interviewing the doctor

Doctors are nervous about being interviewed by prospective patients. Caring doctors do it but it is all rather new to them. Do not be pushy and aggressive. If you are, the doctor may refuse to take you on. Just chat. See what your antennae tell you. If your initial impression is that he is a pain in the butt, then he probably is a pain in the butt. Go elsewhere. If impressions are favourable, join the practice and see what happens.

What if no doctor will take you on?

There are two reasons why a doctor may decline to take you on as a patient:

1. The area in which you live is under-doctored, and all the existing practices are full to bursting. If this is the case, the area will be classified by the FHSA as "open", meaning that new doctors are welcome to set up and may even receive inducements. In the meantime, though, you have a right to a

GP and if none will take you the FHSA will allocate you on a compulsory basis to one of local GPs.

2. You have already been thrown off the lists of several of the local doctors.

Contrary to many patients' fears, it is rare for doctors to throw patients off their lists because they have serious medical problems and are therefore deemed to be too expensive or too much like hard work. If a doctor has removed you for those reasons, he is a skunk and you are better off without him.

If, however, you have been thrown off because you are repeatedly rude and aggressive to doctors and their receptionist then you have only yourself to blame. The FHSA will allocate you a GP but he is only obliged to keep you for ninety days. If he throws you off again, you cannot be re-allocated to him until every GP in the area has had a turn. If you have got yourself into this unhappy situation, your best course of action is to pick the best GP in the area, go and see him, make a clean breast of all your misdemeanours, apologise and ask for a fresh start. You will be taken on again with a clean slate.

Of course, you are very unlikely to take this course of action as you have no insight into the fact that you are poisonous.

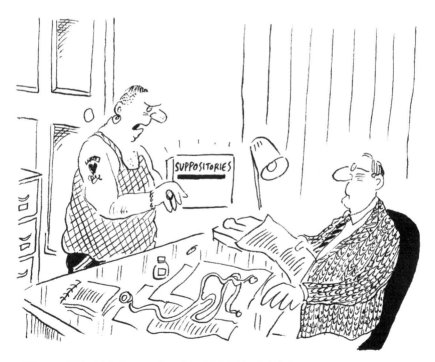

"Course I bin takin 'em – what d'ya think I bin doin, shovin 'em up me arse?"

Sacking a doctor

Patients are inexplicably hesitant about sacking their doctor. This is strange. Most people have no hesitation about sacking a bad solicitor, or a bad accountant or a bad window cleaner. So why not a bad doctor?

It is easy. All you have to do is go and register with another one. Take your medical card with you if you have one (if not the practice will arrange for you to get a new one) and sign on. It is as simple as that.

Patients change doctors for many reasons. No one wants to have a bad doctor, but that is not the usual reason for a move. More likely, there has been a clash of personalities. The doctor's way of dealing with things may not be to your liking. His special interests may not co-incide with the medical needs of your family. The doctor will not be offended if you change. If you are uneasy with the relationship he probably is too and will, with no hard feelings, not be sorry you have left.

Always remember that doctors have an absolute right to sack patients. All they have to do is write to the FHSA as follows:

Dear Sir/Madam

Mr D. Jones, 3 The Avenue, Anytown

Kindly remove this patient from my list forthwith.

Yours faithfully,

DR RUPERT SMITH

That's it. No reason needs to be given. There is no argument. A few days later the patient will get a card form the FHSA telling him that he has been removed from Dr Smith's list.

The patient should be particular aware of the Three Musketeer policy in group practices. Suppose you are registered with Dr Cameron. When he is on holiday you see Dr Finlay a few times, lose your temper with him, and say something you later regret. Or perhaps you do not regret it. It makes no difference. At the next partnership meeting Dr Finlay will tell Dr Cameron that he cannot cope with you and Dr Cameron will remove you from his list. Even if he does not particularly want to. That is the practice policy. All for one and one for all.

Similarly, if you are a patient of a group practice, you have to accept that, particularly when you want an emergency appointment, you may be seen by any of the partners. If you start telling receptionists that you are not prepared to see Dr X or Dr Y, sooner or later you will be removed.

Choosing a Consultant

Asking the gatekeeper

The system in Britain is that the GP acts as the gatekeeper to the NHS.

If you have been admitted to a

hospital as a dire emergency you automatically come under the care of the duty hospital consultant. In all other circumstances you have a choice, and will make that choice in consultation with the GP. In the majority of cases, patients automatically accept the GP's recommendation of the specialist and may not even ask his name. Sometimes patients know of a particular consultant and specifically ask to be referred to him.

Ethically, specialists are not supposed to see patients, either on the NHS or privately, without a referral from the GP. Most will bend the rules and see patients privately without a referral letter and then write to the GP and say what has happened. GPs do not like this. It is hypocrisy. Try to get into the same consultant's NHS outpatients without a referral letter. It may be difficult enough to get in with one!

Some patients get angry with the system. They feel it is a restrictive practice, a closed shop, which prevents them seeing the specialist of their choice. This is not true. In the first place, no sensible GP will decline to refer a patient who insists on being referred, and if he does then the patient can always change doctors. In the second place, and this is the most important reason, the system is there to protect and help the patient, not to hinder him.

The GP is an educated consumer of specialist care. He will first make sure that the specialist matches the problem. The patient may think that Mr Smooth is the best and most charming consultant in the world, but if he is a general surgeon, it is not practical to take a gynaecological problem to him. You waste the cost of the consultation and still have to see someone else.

The GP also knows who are the sensible, ethical and competent specialists. An address on Harley Street or Wimpole Street, three green leather arm chairs and a Sloane Ranger secretary may be very seductive, but means nothing. The only qualification for rooms on Harley Street is the ability to pay the rent.

The Inverse Prejudice Law

We have already discussed the kind and degree of prejudice that is prevalent in the NHS. The Ruperts of this world do well. The fact that a Rupert has reached the exalted heights of a consultant appointment may say more about golf handicaps and goat-shagging than medical abilities.

The astute GP uses his knowledge of prejudice to assess the capability of consultants. Promotion is more difficult for women; they have to be better than their male colleagues to get the same jobs. Similarly, foreign graduates must be better than British; black doctors must be better than brown who must be better than white.

So if you need an operation, apply the inverse prejudice law. The specialist you want is a black, female consultant general surgeon from a working-class background. She will be brilliant. But you will not find her in Britain.

Consultant Quality Control

The conscientious GP considers the following four factors before referring private patients to a consultant:

1. Safety

Do the consultant's patients suffer more than their fair share of complications after surgery? In other words, does he keep cocking it up? If so, the GP will stop using him.

2. Good communication

There is a legal saying that 'Justice must not only be done, it must be seen to be done'. The same is true in medicine. Good doctors communicate with each other. The specialist who never writes to the GP is doing the patient a disservice and may even be dangerous.

3. Morality

Are his criteria for operating the same for NHS patients as they are for private patients? Go to the wrong specialist privately and you'll get the operation whether or not you need it.

4. Fair deal for NHS patients

There is an unspoken contract between GPs and specialists to whom they refer privately that the specialist offers a fair deal to NHS patients. If the specialist is always seeing private patients and leaving NHS patients to the juniors, the discriminating GP will stop referring both groups of patients. This is a question of morality. If you can afford full private health care, you may say 'What care I about the common folk, I go privately.' So be it. But just wait until your insurance runs out, or you retire, or you get a condition that is not covered by your policy.[1]

No *patient* is in a position to make a judgement on the four criteria above. Sensible patients listen to their GP's recommendations. A minority will not. They insist on seeing a specialist who has been recommended by the greengrocer, or whose name they have heard on the radio, or who uses a particular private hospital they like because the food is good. These people are sad. They often have personality problems. They treat their GPs like secretaries not doctors. They move from specialist to specialist getting disease-oriented and non-holistic treatment by charming but often sub-standard doctors. They are a truly pathetic sight when, as it always does, their private cover runs out and they have to rely on the NHS.

[1] Read the small print. There are lots and lots of them.

HOSPITALS
AND HOW TO SURVIVE THEM

When to Avoid Them

The Wrong *Time*

Always have your acute illness between ten o'clock in the morning and four o'clock in the afternoon on any weekday except Friday. If you must choose Friday, make sure it is before midday. Friday afternoon is dangerous. POETS[1] day applies more in medicine than in other professions.

From ten until four, there is a full range of medical and back-up staff. Outside these hours, the hospital becomes a ghost town. The experienced doctors go home from where they may be available on-call. All the laboratory staff are unavailable except in dire emergencies, and even then they decline to come in unless the request is made by a senior registrar or consultant.

[1] Piss Off Early, Tomorrow's Saturday

Casualty is staffed by one lonely, tired and unsupervised SHO. There may be a general medical and general surgical registrar on site, but the registrars in other specialities are at home. Calling in a more senior doctor at night or weekend does not show medical machismo. Juniors who do it can expect a bad reference: "lacking in confidence" or "still inexperienced".

Junior doctors learn their trade at nights and weekends when, unsupervised, they treat patients with serious illness. Out-of-hours surgery is particularly dangerous. The surgeon is inexperienced, there are no proper back-up facilities on site, and the boss is on the golf course. He is carrying a bleep or a mobile telephone but does not expect them to go off.

Most patients admitted as an emergency who need surgery could be stabilised, treated conservatively until the working week starts, and then operated on by fresh, experienced doctors with proper back-up facilities.

Why is this not done? Surgical registrars do not like to postpone operations. Routine Monday morning operating lists would be disturbed. The consultant would be unimpressed. Above all, they would not be showing medical machismo.

The Wrong *Month*

Seafood and hospitals have one thing in common: the former should be avoided if there is not an "r" in the month, the latter if there is not a "k" in the month.

The wise patient will fight shy of February and August. Junior hospital doctors change jobs once or twice a year and the changeover occurs in those two months. On the last day of January, the experienced obstetric SHO saves the life of a baby suffering from foetal distress by doing an efficient and timely forceps delivery. The following day, he turns into the paediatric SHO, takes over the care of the same baby in the Special Care Baby Unit, and, through inexperience, mismanages it.

The registrar has more experience but may not be available. Job-change day means a different room, a different bleep and possibly a different hospital. He may be late back from holiday, or be suffering from a hangover after last night's leaving party.

This hiatus in the continuum of knowledge lasts four to six weeks and occurs twice a year like clockwork.

Avoid it.

The Wrong *Illness*

The art of surviving hospital revolves around having the right illness. It is unwise, sometimes dangerous, to have the wrong one.

The wrong illness includes all conditions that the doctors find boring. Boring illnesses are ones which present no diagnostic challenge, like psoriasis, or ones that cannot be effectively treated, like bad colds, or ones that are both diagnostically unchallenging and untreatable, like strokes.

In the adjacent table is a classification of some common illnesses. Study it carefully and make sure that next time you are ill you choose an illness which will stimulate the doctors and increase the possibility of rational treatment.

The classification only applies to patients under sixty-five. Over that age no illness is fascinating. Over seventy-five, all illness is boring and is dealt with by geriatricians.

Medical students learn to diagnose, treat and cure illness. No-one at medical school ever tells them that some illnesses do not get better; that sometimes patients do not respond to treatment. No-one *ever* tells them that patients die. Life is a temporary and somewhat dangerous position. All patients die eventually; and most of them die in hospital. This is not covered by the medical text books.

Each and every doctor who has ever practised medicine will tell you about the first patient they treated for acute left ventricular failure (LVF) following a heart attack.

They are called to Casualty at three o' clock in the morning to find an elderly and distressed old lady. She is in severe pain; she is short of breath, foaming and bubbling at the mouth; her pulse is weak; her blood pressure is unrecordable. The house officer has been called rather than the registrar because the nurses know she is going to die. They have already labelled her as NFR – 'Not for Resuscitation'.

The house officer does his best. He injects the time-honoured cocktail of drugs. One of the drugs is morphine which immediately relieves the patient's distress. She falls into a deep sleep. She is hardly breathing. Her blood pressure is still unrecordable. She is shipped off to crumble corner. The doctor goes back to bed.

Next morning as he walks onto the ward, he hears a very bad tempered women shouting at the nurses, "I will not eat toast without my teeth. Someone has stolen them. I shall write to the Queen. Where are my teeth?"

The old lady has survived. The house officer is immensely gratified. He has saved a life. He has read about the treatment, but never really believed it would work. But it did. He has treated his first LVF.

The next time, or the time after, or the time after that, it will not work. He will add more drugs. The patient will still deteriorate. He will call the registrar who will decline to come saying, "Look, you have done all the right things; stop getting your knickers in a twist. Go and have a pint." The house officer will be upset. He may cry; in private, if he is wise.

Classification of Illnesses

Fascinating	Dull	Boring
All transplants	Varicose veins	Strokes
Bleeding orifices	Diabetes	Rheumatoid arthritis
Cancer with an unknown primary [1]	Skin disease	Osteoarthritis
Heart attacks	Prostate trouble	Multiple sclerosis
Pneumonia	Period pains	Chronic neurological problems [2]
Broken bones	Cancer with a known primary	All adult psychiatry
Arterial blockages	Epilepsy	Bed-wetting
Gut obstructions	Constipation	Coughs and colds
Asthma	Contraceptive problems	Ingrowing toenails

[1]   'Hunt the Primary' is a favourite medical game – but it is better to travel than arrive

[2]   Unless the patient is a physics professor

As he goes through his career he will learn not to show emotion; to appear impervious to suffering. But it will affect him. He will adopt all sorts of psychological strategies, some conscious, some unconscious, to deal with the stress and anguish.

Medical schools offer no training about dealing with personal mental stress. Medical machismo does not acknowledge it. The doctor may start drinking heavily. He will crack appallingly sick jokes about illness and suffering. One way or another he will sublimate his stress.

His inability to cope with chronic and incurable illness prejudices the way in which he deals with them. The patient he cannot help is sidelined. He begins to classify illness as treatable and untreatable; as interesting and boring. He begins to define "crumble".

Consultants are not immune. They still feel the anguish but can cover it up better. Their sublimation techniques are so sophisticated that they may no longer realise that they are covering up. The astute patient learns to read the consultant. He can even choreograph the consultant's movements round the bed by the way he answers questions. How is it done?

Doctors need to be constantly reassured that they are helping patients. In normal day-to-day conversation, the question "How are you?" is rhetorical, requiring the standard "Fine, fine, and you..." before the main purpose of the conversation is broached. Anyone attempting to answer the question honestly is naive and boring.

The patient might assume that a doctor asking "How are you?" is making a genuine request for details of the patient's state of health. Nothing could be further from the truth. If a doctor wants some specific information about your health he will ask you a specific question like "Do you get rectal bleeding?" Such questions may be answered honestly and succinctly.

When a doctor asks "How are you?" the appropriate answer is "Fine, fine thank you", just like it is with anyone else. But for different reasons. The doctor is not just trying to make polite conversation. The question he is really asking is, "Since I started treating your medical condition are you beginning to feel better?" He does not know how to cope with a negative answer. If he is prone to paranoia, as most doctors are, he will regard a negative answer as a personal criticism of his ability. He will not know how to cope.

And so, on the ward round, if you want to make the consultant dance, when he asks, "How are you?" reply with a mixture of positive and negative answers. After a positive reply such as "Fine, very well" he will advance towards you, maintaining eye contact; he will sit on the side of the bed and shake hands. As he approaches, add "But I'm still in pain from..." and he will retreat immediately.

A negative reply along the lines of "Not so good, actually" makes the consultant take a step backwards, break eye contact with you, turn to the house officer and ask him a question like "What is the serum rhubarb?"

If you feel sorry for him, you can easily add, "But so much better than last week..." so that he can approach again. If the you persist with negative

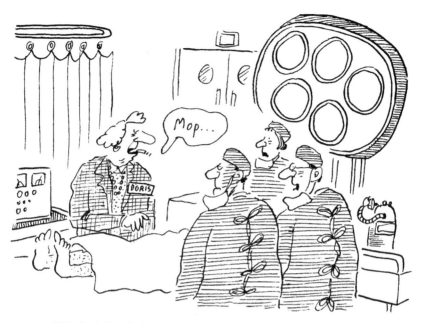

"Oh God, there's been another cock-up with the changeover."

answers he will move on to the next bed, having told the boys to repeat test X,Y or Z.

The Hierarchy Game

Always start at the top if you can. Unfortunately, in hospitals you can't. Within each hospital there is a rigid hierarchy of doctors and nurses. The consultant is at the top and the triage nurse at the bottom. All levels have to be survived before the game is won by meeting the consultant. Some patients never meet the consultant. They are called NHS patients. Patients found cheating by trying to skip a level will be heavily penalised.

Some fall at the first hurdle by failing to arrive safely at the hospital, for the first member of the hierarchy is met in the ambulance. He is:

The Paramedic

The old-fashioned ambulance man was the Dixon of Dock Green of the health service: solid, reliable, calm and sensible. He was far better than doctors at the initial treatment of trauma but never lost sight of his primary function which was to get the seriously-injured patient to hospital alive and as soon as possible. The paramedic is a different beast altogether. He has had a little training in medicine; he has been given machines and drugs to play with. Patients with heart attacks are no longer rushed to hospital. There is delay while the paramedics do ECGs and try to put up drips. They make exotic diagnoses of cardiac problems and initiate treatment. It is interesting to compare the readiness of paramedics and the reluctance of doctors to treat cardiac arrhythmias. A medical houseman with five years training is too nervous to treat them without advice from a senior colleague. Six months later he has the confidence to treat them himself, and does so on many occasions. Six years later, when he is an experienced registrar, and really understands the drugs, he finds he uses them more sparingly. Cardiac drugs are often more dangerous than the conditions they purport to treat. Paramedics can never gain this sort of experience.

At the major road traffic accident, or train crash, the paramedics are invaluable. At the home of the patient with an acute medical problem, they are more dangerous than casualty officers.

Patients surviving the paramedics, and reaching the hospital, next meet:

The Triage Nurse

Triage is a system for categorising emergency admissions which is of particular use when working in a war zone or a disaster area. Patients are divided into one of three groups:

Moribund
Although alive their injuries are so catastrophic that they have little chance of survival and so it is not worth spending any time on them. They are tucked away in a quiet corner to die out of sight.

Seriously ill but treatable
With good care they will survive.

Trivial illness
They can be sent home without treatment and told to buy an elastoplast.

One day someone told the nursing and administrative managers that triage worked well in Vietnam so they decided it would be good for the NHS. No-one told them the NHS is not a war zone.[1]

Casualty departments now have a triage nurse to screen admissions. She will prioritise three patients who present simultaneously with, say, a splinter in a thumb, a sprained ankle and bleeding piles. Sterling work.

At best it is melodramatic nonsense. At worst it is fatal. Nurses are not trained to diagnose and they regularly misinterpret the importance of symptoms. A child with a bit of a temperature and a rash is classified as not urgent and put in a cubicle to die of meningococcal meningitis, whereas a business man with a nose bleed is whisked straight into a treatment room.

Patients surviving the triage nurse next meet:

---

[1] It may be a disaster area

The Casualty Officer

Casualty officers are SHOs. They have been qualified for a minimum of twelve months and are probably in their first post-registration job. They are about twenty-four years old and they are pleased with themselves because this is the first job in which they are allowed to function autonomously as doctors.

As yet, most of them will not have decided on a career. A casualty job is essential for those wanting to be surgeons, a great asset for future GPs and no bad thing to have on your CV for any career. It's a good place to pass time.

Many patients with minor illnesses no longer go to their family doctor but instead go to the hospital where they can see someone in a white coat. They can tell that hospital doctors are cleverer than GPs because they wear white coats. They are real doctors.

Casualty officers are the front end, the business end, of the hospital. They are also the most inexperienced and dangerous doctors in the NHS. Even if they intend to be GPs they have nearly three years of further postgraduate training to complete.

And yet, inexperienced as they are, they make decisions about who is admitted and who is sent home. They order X-Rays and ECGs and interpret and act upon them without assistance. X-Rays taken at the request of casualty officers are checked the next day by the radiologists so that those patients who have fractures that have been missed can be recalled if they are still alive.

Casualty SHOs can always call on the registrars in the various specialities for advice, but are not obliged to do so. Too many requests for help does not show medical machismo. If through luck or judgement the casualty officer decides a patient has a problem that requires admission, he will call the registrar in the appropriate speciality.

The Registrar

Registrars must be at least two years post-qualification and often much more. A surgical registrar about to become a senior registrar may have been qualified for ten years and have taken and passed the FRCS more years ago than he cares to remember. He will be aged anything between twenty-four and thirty-four.

Casualty officers are the bane of the registrar's life. If they are nervous and are forever asking for help they are ridiculed. "Wants to know which hand to wipe his arse with now. Ho! Ho! Ho!".

If they go to the other extreme and send everyone home they will be much celebrated, plied with beer in the residents' bar, and known as 'Killer' behind their backs. Doctors known as 'Killer' have high levels of medical machismo.

The registrar confirms or overrules the casualty officer's decision about admission. The way his decision goes depends on several factors:

1. The bed state - is the ward nearly full? Should the bed be kept for someone who is *really* ill?

2. Does the registrar trust the casualty officer?

3. What's on television.

If the bed state is good, or the casualty officer is reliable, or if there is something good on television, the registrar will accept the admission without getting out of his chair, and tell the casualty officer to call the house officer to clerk the patient in.

It is only when the ward is full and the registrar may want to send the patient home that he actually goes to Casualty himself to see the patient. And if there was something good on television and, having examined the patient, he decides that the complaint is trivial he will bollock the casualty officer for wasting his time. He leaves Casualty telling the Sister to "put that bloody cas officer in the charismatron for an hour".

Patients always survive the registrar and if they are to be admitted now go on to meet:

The House Officer

The house officer is aged twenty-three and has been qualified for many minutes. The patient's chances of surviving the house officer are better than the chances of surviving the Casualty Officer, but are still low. The house officer is less dangerous because he is more humble and knows

that he is ignorant. He is unlikely to try any dangerous manoeuvres, such as treating the patient.

He is really a clerical officer, a booking clerk. He takes the routine medical history from the patient and then examines him from head to foot. If he is an efficient house officer he will insert a finger into the patient's bottom. He does this slowly, cautiously and, unlike his more experienced registrar, he does not wiggle it about very much. This is because as yet he does not know what he is feeling for. The whole business is a voyage of discovery. The patient who is being admitted with a dislocated shoulder wonders why this is necessary but does not like to question someone in a white coat. It is necessary because doctor says it is necessary and doctor has medical machismo.

When he has finished the history and examination the house officer makes a diagnosis and orders some investigations. The number of investigations he orders is inversely proportional to the number of days he has been qualified. It has not yet occurred to him that every test he requests generates a piece of paper which he has to file in the notes. At the beginning of the year the registrar will be taking the piss from him for doing an excessive number of tests; by the end of the year he will be saying, "For God's sake do some investigations. We have to have something to show the boss."

The patient is then dispatched to the ward to await the outcome of the investigations. These will be presented by the houseman to the registrar and a treatment plan instituted. All must be ready for the patient to meet:

The Consultant

The patient may not meet the consultant at all. His chances of meeting him are increased if:

1. He has at any stage seen him privately.

2. He has an interesting condition. The definition of an interesting condition is a condition which the consultant finds interesting.

3. The patient is admitted two to three days before the ward round. If it is longer than that he may already have been cured by the juniors and sent home.

4. The juniors *want* him to meet the consultant. If the juniors feel they have dealt particularly well with the patient, they will deliberately prolong his admission until the ward round so that they can have a mutual preening session. Alternatively, if they have cocked-up on something, they will make sure the patient misses the consultant by arranging for him to be in X-Ray or physiotherapy at the crucial moment.

The consultant ward round is the major ceremonial event of the week:

The ward is tidied. The senior Sister makes sure she is available. The junior doctors assemble all the investigations and information about each patient and rehearse presenting it in a fluid and articulate manner.

Patient mood varies between anxious expectation and naked fear. They have the comforting illusion that the consultant is in constant contact with his team and is familiar with the details of their illness.

In fact, the consultant has never heard of the patient until the houseman presents a summary of the salient points in Sister's office. That presentation goes something like this:

> "Bed 1, 54 year old infarct. Had a clot buster, not in failure, can go home. Bed 2, 70 year old stroke, dense left hemi, relies not interested, trying to bounce him to the gerries. Bed 3, 56 year old diabetic with pneumonia, getting better. Interesting X-Ray."

Patients have a geographical location on the ward, an age, a disease and a best guess as to how long they can occupy the bed. Patients do not have names. If they are lucky, they have an interesting investigation.

When the round starts, Sister will introduce the patient. The consultant will sit on the bed and shake hands with the patient.

It's easy to be a consultant. Anyone can play. Put an ear-to -ear grin on your face. Refer to the chart overleaf and choose any one expression from each column. Put them together.

No medical knowledge is required. The only original thought involves choosing the correct diagnosis for column three. If you are in difficulties an almost subliminal pause will allow the houseman to prompt. If this strat-

The Consultant Ward Round Game

1	2	3	4
Good morning	my dear		You're doing very well and I think we can let you go home
Good afternoon	old chap	Now you seem to have had a spot of bother with . . .	
		[insert medical condition e.g.	or
Nice to meet you	young man	*"heart attack" "stroke" etc.]*	You're doing very well and I will see you next week.
Hello, there	young lady		

egy is adopted then the following phrase should be added; "Of course, of course, just testing the boys, eh?" followed by a wink at the patient.

Routine consultant conventions should be understood:

- Only patients over seventy are described as "young".

- All patients are doing "very well".

- Those patients who are to be seen "next week" are very ill and may not, due to circumstances beyond their control, be available to be seen next week.

The consultant rarely examines the patient other than a ritual touch of the chest with the stethoscope. He is not an examining doctor, or not on NHS patients at any rate. The non-examining rule is waived if there are medical students present. Then there will be at least one examination carried out to impress the boys and girls. The examination will be preceded by the usual ritual humiliation of a student. Let us say that Kevin has just presented the patient.

The boss will ask Kevin if he has done a rectal examination. Kevin has not done one. The boss knows that. Medical students do not do rectal examinations on patients unless they are anaesthetised on an operating table.

"Oh dear, oh dear" says the boss, "If we don't put our finger in it we may put our foot in it, isn't that right, Sister?" Unlike the patient, Sister knows what is coming and produces the consultant's rectal examination tray. When a junior hospital doctor does a rectal examination, he pulls a spare plastic glove out of one pocket of his white coat, a nearly empty tube of KY Jelly from the other pocket, and before the patient can say "uphill gardener" the examination is done. He pinches a tissue from the patient's bedside locker, wipes the bum and chucks the soiled glove in the bin by the locker where the patient's six-year old daughter will find it at visiting time.

The consultant rectal examination is a splendid, choreographed work of art. Sister produces the rectal tray with a flourish. A pair of individually wrapped gloves lies on top.

"Size seven, sister?"

"Size seven, sir"

The consultant dons the gloves and holds out an index finger. Sister squirts a sliver of KY onto the outstretched finger.

"Just turn onto your left side,
old chap, and slip your
trousers down."

The whole ward round assembles around the business end of the bed. The consultant is now addressing the bottom just as he addresses the Haggis on Burns night.

"Rectal examinations can only be
done on your knees."

So saying he kneels on the floor and inserts his index finger into the patient's rectum, right up to the knuckle. He bends forwards and backwards moving the finger in a one hundred and eighty degree circle. The digit is then withdrawn.

"Examine the stool for blood."

The faeculent finger is held in the air for general inspection. Sister wipes the patient's bottom, but the consultant stops her pulling the pyjama trousers up again.

"Just a minute, old chap. You
don't mind if my assistants just
repeat the examinations do
you? We all have to learn."

The patient who was not asked whether he minded the first examination is too speechless to reply. In any case, he is doing his bit for medical education.

The question you, dear reader, must answer is whether you prefer to have multiple rectal examinations done by medical students on an open ward round when you are conscious, and notionally consenting, or whether you would rather have them done when you are anaesthetised and unconsenting.

At the end of the ward round there is an air of relaxation. The boss is on his way back to Harley Street. The juniors are having coffee with Sister. The patients are feeling relieved to have found out that they are all doing well.

DAVID'S HEART ATTACK
A Conducted Tour
of the Hospital

Having now met the team, let us see how a patient admitted as an emergency gets on with them all.

The emergency admission we shall consider is that of a fifty-one year old stockbroker who we shall call David Smith. David has never had a day's illness in his life. He is two stone overweight. He drinks a bottle and a half of wine a day. He tells people he stopped smoking twelve years ago, except for the odd cigar. In fact he smokes ten Slim Panatelas a day. He is concerned about the lack of exercise and has bought a rowing machine on which he now exercises vigorously and inappropriately.

Despite his lifestyle he knows he is fit. How does he know? Because his firm pays £400 a year for him to go to a private health company, CREAM, for a complete medical check up. He has done this every year since he was forty. Each time he has a thorough physical examination, a battery of blood tests, an ECG and more recently an exercise test on a treadmill. There have been one or two minor abnormalities on the blood tests, and he always gets a letter from the screening company which makes some recommendations about his lifestyle (see opposite). It was after the last letter that he went out and bought the rowing machine.

David saw his family doctor a few weeks ago and was given all the same advice as he got from CREAM but, as the advice was free, he ignored it. He is immensely pleased with his so-called normal cardiac screening, and regards it as his licence to abuse his body for another year.

And so, come the day. It is lunch time. He is into his third glass of wine and second Panatela and is discussing the Eurobond market with a colleague when quite suddenly he experiences a gripping, tight pain in the chest. He has never had anything like this before. The pain spreads up to his jaw and feels like toothache. He starts to sweat. He becomes short of breath. His heart races.

David is having his first heart attack and he knows it.

He does not complain when his colleague calls an ambulance. He sits in his chair, frightened. The paramedic ambulance arrives twenty minutes later. He is given oxygen to breath and an aspirin to swallow, and an ECG is recorded there and then in the pub.

David is reassured by the paramedics. He does not realise that the first half hour of the heart attack is statistically the most dangerous period. The best course of action would be for the ambulance to get him to hospital as quickly as possible for further treatment, but the paramedics have to do an ECG first. They do not understand it but it is jolly impressive doing it in a pub; if there are some funny heart beats on it, they will give David some drugs; they do not understand those either but understanding is not on the agenda. Medical machismo is.

If David survives long enough for the paramedics to finish playing doctors they will take him to one of the hospitals that has not had its emergency services closed by the Govern-

What the letter said:

CREAM
The Villas Centre, Hackney

Dear Mr Smith,

It was good to meet you at the Centre last week. I enclose our full report including copies of all the investigations we carried out. With your consent the report has also been sent to your family doctor who will be able to advise you in more detail about the findings.

We agreed that you are a stone and a half overweight and that you should take action to reduce this. You have a busy but sedentary job and it would be helpful to take more exercise.

You smoke two small cigars a day and should really try and stop this altogether. You drink about twenty-five units of alcohol a week and as you know the it accepted recommendation is that you should not exceed twenty-one units. Your cholesterol is a little high at 6.3 mmol/litre but should come down when you lose weight.

The cardiac tracing and exercise test have been reported by our cardiological consultant and I am glad to say they are entirely normal.

I look forward to seeing you next year.

Yours sincerely,

Dr Gillian Nogood MB BS LRCP
MRRCS MRCGP DRCOG

What the letter really meant:

CORPORATE RIP-OFF
EXECUTIVE & MEDICAL SCREENING
The Villas Centre, Hackney

Dear Mr Smith,

I saw sixty executives last week and I hardly remember you. I've sent a copy of all the bumph to your GP but he won't read it and may well chuck it in the bin as it clogs up the notes.

You are a fat bastard. You stink of cigars and I don't believe you only smoke two a day but that's your problem isn't it. You admit to twenty-five units of alcohol a week. Ho! Ho! Ho! Because you are fat, your cholesterol is up. You can try and get it down if you like but in view of your general lifestyle you might as well fart in a thunderstorm.

The cardiac tracing and exercise test have been reported by our cardiological consultant as normal. He knows it is not of much value but we do not pay him to tell you that. This investigation always impresses the punter but you still could have a heart attack tomorrow. Tough!

I hope to God I will have got a proper job by next year instead of doing this dreary screening but if I am still here I will be happy to take another £400 off your company. Not that I see much of it.

Yours sincerely,

Dr Gillian Nogood MB BS LRCP
MRRCS MRCGP DRCOG

ment. If they can find one.

On arrival, he is met by the triage nurse. The paramedics tell her it is a heart attack and even she recognises the seriousness of that problem. The casualty officer arrives, puts a cannula into a vein in the back of David's hand and attaches him to a monitor. He is given an injection for the pain and then attached to a drip which contains something to dissolve clots. The registrar who was watching 'Pebble Mill at One', accepts the admission of a "51-year old MI not in failure". The medical houseman arrives.

He looks younger than David's daughter and has three goes at taking some blood from the arm that is not attached to the drip. At this stage David asks if it makes any difference that he has private health insurance. The houseman scowls, tells him it is up to him how he spends his money, and disappears.

David is moved to the coronary care unit. He is attached to a cardiac monitor and becomes obsessed with the regular beep beep sound. He spends two days on the unit because he has occasional irregularities of his heart rate. This settles and he is moved to an ordinary ward. On day three, having already offended the house officer, he now offends the senior registrar by saying that he has private insurance and would like to see the consultant.

The consultant ward round is not for two more days. However, the ward Sister, who is a crawler, telephones the private secretary and that evening the consultant arrives on the ward unannounced. This angers his junior staff. Diplomatic consultants never, ever do ward rounds without bleeping the houseman. It is just not cricket.

He has a chat with David and gets him moved over to the private ward where he spends another week. This is entirely unnecessary but makes David feel better and makes the consultant and the hospital feel richer. He is sent home by the consultant with an appointment for a follow-up exercise test.

The medical side of the admission has been dealt with appropriately, but because he was in the private ward and was not discharged by the NHS team he has missed out on all the usual advice about lifestyle. Both he and his wife are frightened that sexual intercourse may be dangerous. Their sex life, which was active, stops abruptly and never recovers. The consultant believes it is impertinent to discuss this sort of question unless asked, and he knows that patients do not want to discuss it, as they never ask. The junior doctors would have advised about it as a matter of routine.

Private medical cover is great for varicose veins and bunions but does not work for acute emergencies. Prudent patients do not mention private health insurance to junior hospital doctors.

IS YOUR DOCTOR TELLING THE TRUTH?

The Benevolent Despot

"Before you tell the 'truth' to the patient, be sure you know the 'truth', and that the patient wants to hear it."

RICHARD CLARKE CABOT
(1863-1939)

Traditionally, British doctors have always believed that a patient's diagnosis was none of his business. It was better for him to be kept in the dark. This attitude is no longer widespread, but is still found amongst older members of the profession.

How different it is in the USA. There the doctor comes straight to the point. "George, you have a malignant cancer in your gullet and there is an eighty per cent chance it is going to kill you within a year." American doctors genuinely believe it is right to be up-front, but are also scared of litigation. If they make light of a condition, the patient or his family may sue when it turns out to be more serious than they were originally advised.

One of the British patient's greatest fears is that his doctor is going to lie to him, or hold back part of the truth. There is justification for this fear. Although doctors rarely lie directly, an enormous amount of flannel and subterfuge is used to disguise the seriousness of a diagnosis and to avoid having to confront the patient with the facts of his impending death.

The problem is compounded by the patient. Everyone says, "Oh, yes, when my turn comes, I want to know, I want the truth." When their time does come, they will start to ask questions, but at the last minute back off. Subconsciously they conspire with the doctor, who is equally keen to avoid a direct and unpleasant prognosis, to take refuge in a comforting half-truth.

Imagine a seventy-two year old man, George Adams. He is an intelligent retired businessman. He has been with his doctor for over twenty years and trusts him. He was a heavy smoker until three years ago. He started to cough up blood. The Chest X-Ray showed a cancer of the left lung. It was towards the middle of the chest and inoperable. He has had a course of radiotherapy which has stopped the blood in his sputum. He feels well at present but is losing weight. He goes to his GP for a check up. The GP has just finished examining him.

DOCTOR:	"So George, how are you feeling?"
GEORGE:	"Not bad. My wife's really worried that I'm not putting on weight." [1]
DOCTOR:	"Are you eating?" [2]
GEORGE:	"Yes, very well"
DOCTOR:	"Any pain?"
GEORGE:	"Not really. Hurts a bit when I cough but nothing else."
DOCTOR:	"When is the specialist seeing you again."
GEORGE:	"He was very happy. He doesn't need to see me again." [3]
DOCTOR:	"Oh!"
	pause
GEORGE:	"We were thinking of going to France for a holiday." [4]
DOCTOR:	"When are you going?"
GEORGE:	"July. It is all right for me to go, isn't it?"
DOCTOR:	"Yes, yes, get it booked. Go."
GEORGE:	"Am I going to die doctor?" [5]
DOCTOR:	"We are all going to die sometime, George, and you are seventy-two. But obviously a tumour in the lung is serious and . . ."
GEORGE:	*(Cutting in)* "But I responded to the radiotherapy, didn't I? That's got to be good." [6]
DOCTOR:	"It was encouraging."
GEORGE:	"Good, good, well I'll see you next week then doctor. I'm so grateful."
DOCTOR:	"See you then, George. Any problems give me a ring. And George, if there is anything you want to know, you only have to ask."
GEORGE:	"Thanks doc." [7]

1. Male patients frequently say their wife is worried about something. This means they are worried about it but do not like to make a fuss.

2. Patients with incurable cancer lose weight. Feeding "the crab" never works.

3. Radiotherapists treating lung cancer usually give one course of treatment and do not bother to offer a follow-up appointment as there is nothing more they can do. They do not tell the patient how serious the condition is. When the patient is not offered a follow-up appointment he either thinks he has had it, which in this case is true, or sometimes thinks it means he has been cured, which is never true.

4. George floats the idea of a holiday to test the water. The doctor says, yes - if you are quick.

5. George summons up the nerve to ask the direct question which the doctor shamefully flannels.

6. Both are relieved to have moved on from death, and take mutual refuge in discussing the effect of radiotherapy.

7. George leaves feeling reassured. The doctor has not actually said he is going to die of the condition and stressed at the end of the consultation that he will always answer questions truthfully.

There are conversations like this going on every day in GP's surgeries throughout the country. George and his doctor are both intelligent men and are playing a psychological game. The doctor knows that George will die in a few months time, perhaps a year if he is lucky. George knows that lung cancer is serious, and the rational, businessman part of his brain knows he has not been cured. George is also an optimist and a fighter. He wants to spare his wife and family anguish by protecting them from knowledge of the prognosis. His wife and family are entirely aware of the prognosis, but want to protect George, and so they go along with the charade. This silent conspiracy leads to a falsely jolly environment at home, and prevents the family discussing the things they really want to discuss. The wife will have a prolonged bereavement when George dies as she has not been able to prepare herself by saying goodbye.

The doctor would like to spell out the prognosis but cannot summon up the nerve to do it. George has some important questions he wants to ask about how he is likely to die, and whether the pain, if there is any, can be controlled. He is terrified that as he gets weaker he will become incontinent. He tries to give the doctor the opportunity to talk openly but shears off at the last minute.

Both George and his doctor are as bad as each other as communicators. But it is probably fair to say that neither wanted to talk about the truth and they are to be complimented on avoiding it so elegantly.

Does your Doctor *Know* the Truth?

Life is a precarious and ephemeral condition, and all of us, even health-conscious Americans, are going to leave it sometime. There is no question a doctor dreads more than, "How long have I got?"

When asked the question, the first thing the doctor must do is resist the temptation to look at his watch. Having avoided that trap, the question can be given serious consideration. On an individual basis it is unanswerable with any degree of accuracy. However serious the illness, patients are all different and may defy the statistics. Most doctors who are prepared to answer directly will say something like, "Months rather then years" or "Days rather than weeks", but will always add that they can never be sure. This is not flannel.

Strangely, the doctors who are most likely to be dishonest about prognoses are the cancer specialists: the radiotherapists and oncologists. They are not wilfully dishonest. It is just that they live in a parallel universe on a different planet. On **Planet Cancer**. All people on **Planet Cancer** have ...cancer. They are kept alive for long periods, and sometimes even cured, by the cancer specialists.

When those specialists tell a patient that the outlook is good, remember that they come from a different planet and are not speaking the same language as earth people. Consider a condition like Hodgkin's Disease, which is a malignant cancer of the lymphatics. This disease is fatal if untreated. Over the last forty years advances in radiotherapy and chemotherapy, pioneered by the cancer specialists, mean that with aggressive treatment it can more often than not be cured. It is a young person's cancer.

Take a group of thirty young people, in their late teens, and tell them that they have a condition at a certain stage of development which can be cured in eighty per cent of cases. To the radiotherapist this is a wonderful outlook. And so it may be on **Planet Cancer**. But translate it into Earth language. Six of those thirty teenagers, twenty per cent of them, are going to die notwithstanding the best possible treatment. Is that a good prognosis for a group of teenagers?

Cancer Code - what does the doctor *really* mean?

If you go to the Czech Republic for your holidays and talk to some locals you will find communication difficult. Few speak English, and the problem is compounded by the fact that the Czech word for "Yes" sounds like the English "No". But at least you *know* you are speaking two different languages and can make allowances.

Doctors speak a different language to patients but neither party acknowledges the fact. If communication is to go well, both parties should define their terms. Let us give a few examples of commonly misunderstood words and expressions:

Patients use the word 'cancer' to mean a serious, malignant, probably incurable growth. In fact, a cancer can be malignant or benign (a verruca is a cancer), and a doctor may use the word to denote either type. 'Tumour' sounds less serious to patients but in fact is a synonym for cancer. The words which a doctor has at his disposal to denote a growth that is definitely malignant range from the scientific-sounding to the deceptively friendly: neoplasm, space-occupying lesion, mitotic lesion, crab and Charlie are all words for a malignant growth. Most patients would never guess.

This kind of double-talk isn't helpful. To avoid all doubt, both doctors and patients should agree to talk bout malignant cancers.

The Questions to Ask to Get the Right Answers

Do you really want to know?

First of all, you must be certain that you *want* the right answers; that you are ready to face up to the stark, unadorned truth.

Secondly, remember that no doctor can give you a precise quantification of your life expectancy, whether or not you have a serious illness. He can only quote statistics, and statistics apply to populations not to individuals.

Thirdly, bear in mind that we all have to die of something. To tell an eighty-year old that he has a condition that will kill him within ten years

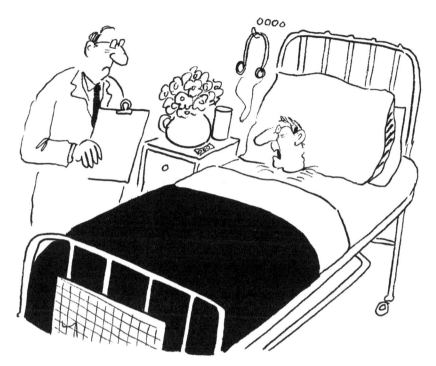

"Give it to me straight Doc, how serious is it?"

is less serious than to tell the same to a fifty-year old. Actuarially, an eighty-year old is not going to live long enough to die of the condition.

The Precise Diagnosis

You cannot get a prognosis unless and until you have a precise diagnosis. Being told you have cancer will not do. You need to have a tissue diagnosis and you need to know the stage the disease has reached.

We have concentrated on malignant cancers so far in this chapter but there are many other non-malignant

conditions which can be just as, or more, serious. People are gung-ho about having heart attacks. They are not perceived as very serious. And yet a third of people who have heart attacks will die from them in the medium term and about half will die from them within ten years. If there are complications after the first attack, such as heart failure, the prognosis is worse.

Clinical Observation

Medical students are encouraged to detect subtle signs of illness. The astute patient who wants to understand his illness will likewise learn to pick up subtle signs from both doctors and nurses and from the hospital environment.

• Bed Position

When you arrive on the ward, note which bed you are allocated. Patients in the bed closest to Sister's desk at the front of the ward have serious and interesting illnesses. During their stay their bed will be moved down the ward towards the day room. This movement means either:

1. They are getting better;

or

2. They are getting worse but their condition has become boring or incurable. All incurable illnesses are boring.

The worst place to be is in a far-flung corner of a medical ward. That is where the strokes live whilst they wait for a bed to come free on the geriatric ward. This is 'crumble corner'. The letters 'NFR' are written on these patients' notes, sometimes even on the end of their beds.

• Eye Contact

Junior doctors do not understand patients who fail to respond to treatment. They get cross, bad-tempered, and avoid eye contact.

Does the houseman look at you when you ask a question?

Any eye contact at all with a consultant is significant. Consultants do not visit crumble corner. They pretend it does not exist. They may glance down to the end of the ward and berate the houseman for allowing the acute beds to be blocked.

A leading London teaching hospital consultant surgeon had one of his acute beds blocked by Patrick, a homeless Irish vagrant, who had been admitted with gangrene in both feet. After a double below-knee amputation he was immobile. He had no family. He was too young even for the geriatricians. There was nowhere for him to go.

After some months, the consultant turned to the houseman and said, "Get rid of that patient. I don't ever want to see him again on my ward."

At three o'clock the next morning, the houseman went on to the ward, arranged for the Night Sister to be distracted, and bundled Patrick into a wheelchair. He took him across the hospital to one of the medical wards. He wrote out a bogus entry in the nursing notes, and popped Patrick into an empty bed.

The nurses fed him; the doctors ignored him, each thinking he was someone else's patient. Patrick happily played along; it was better than the Embankment. It was five weeks before anyone noticed.

The Prognosis

Doctors look at the prognosis of conditions statistically. They consider how many people diagnosed as having a certain condition at a certain stage will be alive in a given number of years. This is the 'X year survival rate'. The 'one year survival rate' and the 'five year survival rate' are commonly quoted. These are statistical concepts that apply to large populations and not to individuals but they are accurate. A knowledgeable bookie would quote on them.

But try to put it in context. Look at the statistics in the table below.

Conclusion: Demanding the Truth

Make an appointment to see the doctor. Tell him immediately that you want an open discussion of your medical condition. Ask specifically for the precise diagnosis, including the staging of the disease if appropriate; ask if you have any recognised adverse complications.

Having established that, ask for the one and five year survival rates for the condition.

If you are still not clear at the end of the consultation, put your questions in writing.

Annual Risk of Death from Various Activities

Smoking ten cigarettes a day	1 in 250
All natural causes aged 40	1 in 850
Any kind of violence or poisoning	1 in 3300
Road traffic accident	1 in 8000
Accident at home	1 in 26,000
Homicide (in UK not USA)	1 in 100,000
Being hit by lightning	1 in 10,000,000

ON DEATH AND DYING

Note: Those of a squeamish disposition should skip the next few pages. We are going to consider what *really* happens when you die.

Is the Patient Dead?

How do you know if someone is dead? Actually, it's pretty easy to tell. Only trained nurses have difficulty in making the diagnosis.

It is not strictly necessary for a doctor to see a body to confirm death. There is a difference between confirming death and issuing a Death Certificate. In the majority of cases, the doctor will want to see the body, particularly if the patient has died at home, so that he is better able to fill in the Death Certificate and also comfort the bereaved. But if, for example, the patient has been seen by the doctor on Saturday morning in the cottage hospital, is over ninety, is terminally ill and unconscious, and is expected to die within a few hours, when he does die early the following morning, it is not essential for the doctor to attend.

Nurses do not understand this. When they suspect death, they will call the doctor. The conversation will go like this:

6.45 a.m. The phone is answered on the third ring.

Sister "Sorry to disturb you before breakfast, Doctor"

Doctor "That's all right. What's the problem?"

Sister "Mr Smith died at four o'clock this morning."

Doctor "Oh dear, poor old boy . . still, a blessed release really."

Sister "When will you come to certify death?"

momentary pause

Doctor "I don't need to. Tell the family to get on with the arrangements and I'll call in to see them this afternoon."

Sister "I can't release the body until you have confirmed that he is dead."

Doctor "Yes you can."

Sister "No I can't. I'm not covered."

Doctor "Is the patient breathing Sister? Does he have a pulse?"

Sister "Doctor, I'm not allowed to say that a patient is dead."

Doctor (wearily) "How long have you been a nurse, Sister?"

Sister "Doctor, you know the regulations. Why do we always have this argument?"

Doctor (resigned) "Alright, alright, I'll pop in this morning. But it's quite unnecessary, you know."

Sister "Can you make sure you get here before nine because the undertaker is arriving then?"

Doctor "How can you call the undertaker if you don't know the patient's dead?"

Sister "See you later."

The doctor arrives at the cottage hospital and goes straight to the patient's bed which is empty. He calls Sister.

Doctor "Where is Mr Smith, Sister?"

Sister "In the mortuary."

Doctor "When did you put him there?"

Sister "Five o' clock this morning."

Doctor "So he's been in the fridge for four hours now?"

Sister "Yes."

Doctor (walking out) "Well, we'll just have to hope he was dead before you put him in, won't we?"

Nurses specialise in this sort of nonsense. It is part of their training.

Notice to Informant

This is the bit that you get to see (page 186). It tells you that the doctor has certified the death of the patient and gives the date.

It does not tell you the cause of death, because that is a secret, for doctors to share with each other, and certainly not something that can be trusted to the likes of you.

The Death Certificate proper is given to you in a sealed envelope but there is nothing to stop you opening it to have a look. If you do, you will see the form that is reproduced on pages 187 and 188.

Your duties are listed at the bottom right of the form together with a stern warning that your bottom may be smacked if you do not comply.

On the reverse side there are details of who is allowed to deliver the certificate to the registrar. It is usually a member of the family, but broadly speaking, anyone can act as informant.

The Death Certificate

This is the bit you usually do not see. You can see it now on page 187. Certification *should* be straightforward, but it is not for two reasons:

1. There are complex rules surrounding certification which no doctor properly understands.

2. Certificates issued in hospitals, the majority, are filled in by a junior doctor who may not have a clue of the real cause of death. Equally, the GP in the home environment, though much more experienced, may not be sure of the cause of death. His main concern is to dream up something plausible that will be legally acceptable and spare the family the trauma of a post-mortem.

All the information on a Death Certificate is used for national

MED A 970855
19

(Form prescribed by the Registration of Births and Deaths Regulations 1987)

NOTICE TO INFORMANT

I hereby give notice that I have this day signed a medical certificate of cause of death of

....

....

Signature ....

Date ....

This notice is to be delivered by the informant to the registrar of births and deaths for the sub-district in which the death occurred.

The certifying medical practitioner must give this notice to the person who is qualified and liable to act as informant for the registration of death (see list overleaf).

DUTIES OF INFORMANT

Failure to deliver this notice to the registrar renders the informant liable to prosecution. The death cannot be registered until the medical certificate has reached the registrar.

When the death is registered the informant must be prepared to give to the registrar the following particulars relating to the deceased:

1. The date and place of death.

2. The full name and surname (and the maiden surname if the deceased was a woman who had married).

3. The date and place of birth.

4. The occupation (and if the deceased was a married woman or a widow the name and occupation of her husband).

5. The usual address.

6. Whether the deceased was in receipt of a pension or allowance from public funds.

7. If the deceased was married, the date of birth of the surviving widow or widower.

THE DECEASED'S MEDICAL CARD SHOULD BE DELIVERED TO THE REGISTRAR

PERSONS QUALIFIED AND LIABLE TO ACT AS INFORMANTS

The following persons are designated by the Births and Deaths Registration Act 1953 as qualified to give information concerning a death:—

DEATHS IN HOUSES AND PUBLIC INSTITUTIONS

(1) A relative of the deceased, present at the death.

(2) A relative of the deceased, in attendance during the last illness.

(3) A relative of the deceased, residing or being in the sub-district where the death occurred.

(4) A person present at the death.

(5) The occupier* if he knew of the happening of the death.

(6) Any inmate if he knew of the happening of the death.

(7) The person causing the disposal of the body.

DEATHS NOT IN HOUSES OR DEAD BODIES FOUND

(1) Any relative of the deceased having knowledge of any of the particulars required to be registered.

(2) Any person present at the death.

(3) Any person who found the body.

(4) Any person in charge of the body.

(5) The person causing the disposal of the body.

*"Occupier" in relation to a public institution includes the governor, keeper, master, matron, superintendent, or other chief resident officer.

MED A 9 7 0 8 5 5
19

Registrar to enter
No. of Death Entry

BIRTHS AND DEATHS REGISTRATION ACT 1953
(Form prescribed by the Registration of Births and Deaths Regulations 1987)

MEDICAL CERTIFICATE OF CAUSE OF DEATH

For use only by a Registered Medical Practitioner WHO HAS BEEN IN ATTENDANCE during the deceased's last illness, and to be delivered by him forthwith to the Registrar of Births and Deaths.

Name of deceased ....

Date of death as stated to me .... day of .... Age as stated to me ....

Place of death ....

Last seen alive by me .... day of ....

1   The certified cause of death takes account of information obtained from post-mortem.

2   Information from post-mortem may be available later.

3   Post-mortem not being held.

4   I have reported this death to the Coroner for further action.

[See overleaf]

Please ring appropriate digit(s) and letter.

a   Seen after death by me.

b   Seen after death by another medical practitioner but not by me.

c   Not seen after death by a medical practitioner.

CAUSE OF DEATH

The condition thought to be the 'Underlying Cause of Death' should appear in the lowest completed line of Part I.

I(a)   Disease or condition directly leading to death† ....

(b)   Other disease or condition, if any, leading to I(a) ....

(c)   Other disease or condition, if any, leading to I(b) ....

II   Other significant conditions CONTRIBUTING TO THE DEATH but not related to the disease or condition causing it. ....

These particulars not to be entered in death register

Approximate interval between onset and death

The death might have been due to or contributed to by the employment followed at some time by the deceased.

Please tick where applicable

†*This does not mean the mode of dying, such as heart failure, asphyxia, asthenia, etc: it means the disease, injury, or complication which caused death.*

I hereby certify that I was in medical attendance during the above named deceased's last illness, **and that the particulars and cause of death above written are true to the best of my knowledge and belief.**

Signature ....

Qualifications as registered by General Medical Council }

Residence ....

Date ....

Complete where applicable

A

I have reported this death to the Coroner for further action. ....

Initials of certifying medical practitioner. ....

B

I may be in a position later to give, on application by the Registrar General, additional information as to the cause of death for the purpose of more precise statistical classification. ....

Initials of certifying medical practitioner. ....

The Coroner needs to consider all cases where:

The death might have been due to or contributed to by a violent or unnatural cause (including an accident);

or the cause of death cannot be identified;

or the death might have been due to or contributed to by drugs, medicine, abortion or poison;

or there is reason to believe that the death occurred during an operation or under or prior to complete recovery from an anaesthetic or arising subsequently out of an incident during an operation or an anaesthetic;

or the death might have been due to or contributed to by the employment followed at some time by the deceased.

LIST OF SOME OF THE CATEGORIES OF DEATH WHICH MAY BE OF INDUSTRIAL ORIGIN

MALIGNANT DISEASES

Causes include:

(a) Skin
- radiation and sunlight
- pitch or tar
- mineral oils

(b) Nasal
- wood or leather work
- nickel

(c) Lung
- asbestos
- nickel
- radiation

(d) Pleura
- asbestos

(e) Urinary Tract
- benzidine
- dyestuff
- chemicals in rubbers
- PVC manufacture

(f) Liver
- radiation

(g) Bone
- radiation
- benzene

(h) Lymphatics and haematopoietic

POISONING

(a) Metals — e.g. arsenics, cadmium, lead

(b) Chemicals — e.g. chlorine, benzene

(c) Solvents — e.g. trichlorethylene

INFECTIOUS DISEASES

Causes include:

(a) Anthrax
- imported bone, bonemeal, hide or fur

(b) Brucellosis
- farming or veterinary

(c) Tuberculosis
- contact at work

(d) Leptospirosis
- farming, sewer or underground workers

(e) Tetanus
- farming or gardening

(f) Rabies
- animal handling

(g) Viral hepatitis
- contact at work

BRONCHIAL ASTHMA AND PNEUMONITIS

(a) Occupational asthma
- sensitising agent at work

(b) Allergic Alveolitis
- farming

PNEUMOCONIOSIS
- mining and quarrying
- potteries
- asbestos

NOTE:—The Practitioner, on signing the certificate, should complete, sign and date the Notice to the Informant, which should be detached and handed to the Informant. The Practitioner should then, without delay, deliver the certificate itself to the Registrar of Births and Deaths for the sub-district in which the death occurred. Envelopes for enclosing the certificates are supplied by the Registrar.

epidemiological research. Unfortunately the information is hopelessly flawed because of the inherent inaccuracies of the system.

An elderly patient who has been fading peacefully at home is likely to be certified as having died of bronchopneumonia, or a heart attack, or a stroke, when there is not a jot of evidence to support those diagnoses, other than a statistical likelihood.

A doctor who has attended a patient during his last illness is obliged to certify the cause of death and no other doctor may do it on his behalf. The doctor himself must decide in a reasonable fashion whether he was in attendance. If he has not seen the patient for a year, the answer if obvious, as it is if he has seen him every day for the last month. The difficulty comes in between. If the doctor has for example been away on holiday he may be asked to certify a death when he has not seen the body nor has he seen the patient alive for over fourteen days. Despite this, he may still be in the best position to certify the death, but will have to report the situation to the coroner, who will decide what further action is necessary.

Earning the 'Ash Cash'

Patients who are to be cremated require a second death certificate, called a Cremation Form. This has to be signed by two doctors, one of whom must be independent. The fee earned for completing it is known in the trade as "Ash Cash" and is at present sixty-four pounds, which is split by the doctors.

If the Death Certificate is sometimes inaccurate, the Cremation Form (see pages 190-193) is a work of pure fiction. Unlike the Death Certificate, it is an absolute requirement that the doctors signing the Cremation Form must see the body and thoroughly examine it. Usually, this means a trip to the undertakers to look in the 'fridge' or open the box. Not a pleasant business and just because doctors do it frequently does not mean they like it. So they skimp. A quick glimpse at the face to confirm identity and that's it. The certified cause of death, say a heart attack, is confirmed. The "examination" performed is inadequate and potentially negligent. If the patient has a machete stuck in his back it will not be noticed or commented on as possibly implicated in the patient's demise.

This disrespect for the procedure is compounded by the inanity of some of the questions. Take the 'Mode of Death' question. This requires the doctor to say whether the mode of death was "syncope, coma, exhaustion, convulsions etc.". No doctor knows how to answer this question. 'Syncope' means cardiac arrest - well, everyone dies of that; you may die *in* a coma, but you hardly die *from* it; what is exhaustion and can it be a mode of death?

The doctors are supposed to meet and talk about the patient. They never meet. A quick telephone call suffices, sometimes not even that. If the patient died at home, the Certificate will be filled in by two GPs in different practices. In hospitals, the consultant pathologists usually monopolise the Part C trade and fill in several a day after a brief chat with the junior doctor. At thirty-two pounds a time, a source of serious income.

190

This confirmatory certificate is NOT required when question 8A of Form B has been answered in the affirmative.

FORM **C.**

CONFIRMATORY MEDICAL CERTIFICATE

(Pursuant to No. 9 of the Cremation Regulations, 1930 and 1952)

The Confirmatory medical certificate in Form C, if not given by the Medical Referee, must be given by a registered medical practitioner of not less than 5 years' standing, who shall not be a relative of the deceased or a relative or partner of the doctor who has given the certificate in Form B.

𝕴, being neither a relative of the deceased, nor a relative or partner of the medical practitioner who has given the foregoing medical certificate, have examined it and have made personal inquiry as stated in my answers to the questions below,:—

(The doctor must see the body of the deceased.)

(4) Each question MUST be answered.

This answer should be 'YES'
1. Have you seen the body of the deceased?

This answer should be 'YES'
2. Have you carefully examined the body externally?

3. Have you made a post mortem examination?

(Additional information requested by Medical Referee)
Has a post mortem examination been performed? | If so by whom?

This answer should be 'YES'
4. Have you seen and questioned the medical practitioner who gave the above certificate?

5. (a) Have you seen and questioned any other medical practitioner who attended the deceased?
(a)................
(b) (Give names and addresses of persons seen and say whether you saw them alone.)
(b)................

6. (a) Have you seen and questioned any person who nursed the deceased during the last illness, or who was present at the death?
(a)................
(b) (Give names and addresses of persons seen and say whether you saw them alone.)
(b)................

7. (a) Have you seen and questioned any of the relatives of the deceased?
(a)................
(b) (Give names and addresses of persons seen and say whether you saw them alone.)
(b)................

8. (a) Have you seen and questioned any other person?
(a)................
(b) (Give names and addresses of persons seen and say whether you saw them alone.)
(b)................

Here insert cause of death:
𝕴 am 𝖘𝖆𝖙𝖎𝖘𝖋𝖎𝖊𝖉 that the cause of death was................

....

and I certify that I know of no reasonable cause to suspect that the deceased died either a violent or an unnatural death or a sudden death of which the cause is unknown or died in such place or circumstances as to require an inquest in pursuance of any Act.

Name ....
(BLOCK CAPITALS)

(Signature) ....
(Address) ....

....

(Date)................

(Tel. No.) ....

Registered Qualifications................

Year of FULL Registration ....

This certificate may only be given by a medical practitioner who has been FULLY REGISTERED with the General Medical Council in this country for at least 5 years.

NOTE:- *These Certificates after being signed by both the medical practitioners must be handed or sent in a closed envelope to*

CREMATION ACTS, 1902 & 1952

Form F.

To be left blank. This Certificate
will be obtained by the Cremation
Authority.

*Required by the Regulations made
by the Secretary of State for the
Home Department, 1930 and 1952.*

Authority to Cremate

Whereas I have satisfied myself in respect of the application made for the Cremation of the remains of the within-named deceased that all the requirements of the Cremation Acts, 1902 and 1952, and of the regulations made in pursuance of those Acts, have been compiled with, that the cause of death has been definitely ascertained and that there exists no reason for any further inquiry or examination.

I accordingly hereby authorise The Superintendent of the

, to cremate the said remains.

(Signature) ....

Medical Referee of

(Date) ....

This form is issued by

No.................................

Forms B C & F

CREMATION ACTS, 1902 AND 1952

Cremation Regulations, 1930, 1952, 1965 and 1985

These Forms are Statutory. All the questions must be answered, therefore, to make the Certificate effective for the purposes of Cremation.

These medical certificates are regarded as strictly confidential. The right to inspect them is confined to the Secretary of State, the Ministry of Health, and the Chief Officer of a Police Force.

CERTIFICATE OF MEDICAL ATTENDANT

𝕴 am informed that application is about to be made for the cremation of the remains of—

FORM **B.**

(1) This form is not to be used in the case of a Coroner's Inquest.

(Name of Deceased)..

(Address) ....

(Occupation or Description) .... (Age)..............

Having attended the Deceased before death, and seen and identified the body after death I give the following answers to the questions set out below:—

(2) NOTE. — The answers to the questions should be as concise as possible. Figures may be used instead of words. All the questions must be answered.

1. On what date, and at what hour, did he or she die?	
2. What was the place where the deceased died? (Give address and say whether own residence, lodging, hotel, hospital, nursing home, etc.)	(If in hospital, date admitted)
3. Are you a relative of the deceased? If so, state the relationship.	
4. Have you, so far as you are aware, any pecuniary interest in the death of the deceased?	
5. (a) Were you the ordinary medical attendant of the deceased? (b) If so, for how long?	(a) .... (b) ....
6. (a) Did you attend the deceased during his or her last illness? (b) If so, for how long?	(a) .... (b) ....

(3) Cases where the deceased was attended by a doctor for less than 24 hours OR where the doctor has not attended within 14 days should be notified to the Coroner.

7. When did you last see the deceased alive? (Say how many days or hours before death.)	
(Additional information requested by Medical Referee) Has the death been notified to the Coroner?	
	(The doctor must see the body after death)
8. (a) How soon after death did you see the body? (b) What examination of it did you make?	(a) .... (b) ....
8A. If the deceased died in a hospital* at which he was an in-patient, has a post-mortem examination been made by a registered medical practitioner of not less than five year's standing who is neither a relative of the deceased nor a relative or a partner of yours and are the results of that examination known to you?	
9. What was the cause of death? I. Immediate cause. Morbid conditions, if any, giving rise to immediate cause (stated in order proceeding backwards from immediate cause).	(a) .... due to (b) .... due to (c) ....
II. Other morbid conditions (if important) contributing to death but not related to immediate cause.	....

IMPORTANT: Pacemakers can cause an explosion if left in a body which is cremated. Radio-active implants are a health hazard.

Please answer the following questions:

i) Has the deceased been fitted with (a) a cardiac pacemaker?   YES/NO
                       (b) A radio-active or other implant?   YES/NO

ii) If the answer to (a) or (b) above is in the affirmative: Has this been removed?   YES/NO

NOTE: CREMATION MAY BE REFUSED IF A PACEMAKER IS NOT REMOVED.

10. *(a)* What was the mode of death? (Say whether syncope, coma, exhaustion, convulsions, etc.)	*(a)* ....
(b) What was its duration in days, hours, or minutes?	*(b)* ....
11. State how far the answers to the last two questions are the result of your own observations, or are based on statements made by others. If on statements by others, say by whom.	
12. *(a)* Did the deceased undergo any operation during the final illness or within a year before death?	*(a)* ....
(b) If so, what was its nature and who performed it?	*(b)* ....
13. By whom was the deceased nursed during his or her last illness? Give names, and say whether professional nurse, relative, etc. If the illness was a long one, this question should be answered with reference to the period of four weeks before the death.)	
14. Who were the persons (if any) present at the moment of death?	
15. In view of the knowledge of the deceased's habits and constitution, do you feel any doubt whatever as to the character of the disease or the cause of death?	
16. Have you any reason to suspect that the death of the deceased was due, directly or indirectly, to *(a)* Violence .... *(b)* Poison .... *(c)* Privation or neglect	Death due directly or indirectly to alcohol has now to be reported to the Coroner.
17. Have you any reason whatever to suppose a further examination of the body to be desirable?	
18. Have you given the certificate required for registration of death? If not, who has?	

𝔍 𝔥𝔢𝔯𝔢𝔟𝔶 ℭ𝔢𝔯𝔱𝔦𝔣𝔶 that the answers given above are true and accurate to the best of my knowledge and belief, and that I know of no reasonable cause to suspect that the deceased died either a violent or an unnatural death or a sudden death of which the cause is unknown or died in such place or circumstances as to require an inquest in pursuance of any Act.

Name .... *(Signature)* ....
(BLOCK CAPITALS)

(Address) .... *(Registered Qualifications)* ....

(Date) .... *(Tel. No.)* .... *Date of registration* ....

NOTE: THE MEDICAL PRACTITIONER WHO SIGNS THE CERTIFICATE MUST HAND OR SEND IT IN A CLOSED ENVELOPE TO THE PRACTITIONER WHO IS TO GIVE THE CONFIRMATION CERTIFICATE, EXCEPT IN A CASE WHERE QUESTION 8A IS ANSWERED IN THE AFFIRMATIVE, IN WHICH CASE THE CERTIFICATE MUST BE SO HANDED OR SENT TO THE MEDICAL REFEREE.

* The term "hospital" as used here means any Institution for the reception and treatment of persons suffering from illness or mental disorder, any maternity home, and any Institution for the reception and treatment of persons during convalescence.

Additional information regarding either of the Certificates may be given here if necessary.

Post-Mortems

Patients silly enough to die without first giving their doctor the information he needs to enter a plausible albeit inaccurate cause of death on the certificate will be the subject of a coroner's post-mortem. This is the final and definitive surgical procedure. It is not done by the coroner. It is farmed out to local pathologists who do five or six a week. More if they are lucky.

Coroner's post-mortems are nothing to do with Marcus Welby MD or Sherlock Holmes. The overwhelming majority of them are totally, utterly monotonous and boring. Just as doctors skimp the examination of the body before filling in the Cremation Form, so pathologists skimp routine post-mortems. An examination that cannot be done properly in under an hour is completed in ten minutes. Once an acceptable cause of death has been found, whole areas of the body are left unexamined; classically the skull is not opened.

Death and Dishonesty

There must be a system in place to investigate suspicious or unexpected deaths. But the present bureaucratic rigmarole is ill-thought out.

It produces a huge income for doctors, income which is too easily earned for work not properly done. The statistics it generates on 'cause of death' are wildly inaccurate. Worst of all, it results in many unnecessary post-mortems, causing anxiety and distress to families of the deceased.

CRAWLING UP YOUR DOCTOR'S NOSE

Heartsink Patients

When a doctor looks at the list of patients for his next clinic or surgery he scans briefly down the names. One or two, or sometimes more if it is not his lucky day, will make him think, or in extreme cases say out loud, "Oh God!"

These are the 'heartsink' patients. They are a mountain on the horizon of the clinic and the doctor will be on edge until he has climbed the mountain and is safely down the other side.

The concept of the heartsink patient originated in general practice, but is familiar to all doctors in all specialities. There are many different types of patient that fit into the category. The wise patient studies the characteristics of the heartsink and avoids them. Here are some recent descriptions:[1]

The dependant clinger

The entitled demander

The manipulative help-rejecter

The self-destructive denier

[1] This classification is described by Carson, Norris & Haworth in The Practitioner 287 (1525): 313-9 April 1993

or

The never-get-betters

The not-one-but-twos

The medico-socially deprived

The wicked manipulators

The sad

or

Black holes

Family complexity

Punitive behaviour

Personal links to the doctor's character

Differences in culture and belief

Disadvantage, poverty and deprivation

Medical complexity

Medical connections

Wicked manipulative and playing games

Secrets

These lists were made by three different doctors. The characterisations are not the product of whim or idle reflection. They are a serious attempt by the GPs to look at areas of strain in the doctor-patient relationship. All doctors get frustrated by patients. But when the relationship breaks down totally it is more often due to the deficiencies of medical training than to the behaviour of the patients

A hundred years ago, people took their problems to the priests or to an old and wise member of the extended family. God has been rumbled; he never came up with the answers; he could not deliver the goods. The elderly members of the extended family have been shunted off to sheltered accommodation or nursing homes where they receive a grudging weekly visit and an annual trip out for Christmas lunch.

The doctor takes over both roles, but has been trained for neither. He is an inadequate god and a dreadful grandmother.

Doctors are problem-solvers. They like to assess, diagnose, treat and cure. That approach has been drummed into them at medical school. When patients bring in their *insoluble* personal, social, sexual and psychological problems, doctors do not know how to cope. They have not been trained for it.

To complicate matters further, patients are aware that the doctor is not the correct person to approach, and so they camouflage the problem behind minor physical complaints. Many doctors, in particular hospital-based ones, conspire with the patient to pretend that the physical problem is the real problem. The doctor offers treatment, maybe a drug, maybe an operation, for the physical symptoms and gets the patient out of the clinic quickly. But the patient will soon be back to offer another physical symptom.

When they are repeatedly faced with insoluble problems, sometimes by difficult, poisonous and manipulative patients, but more often just by

sad people with life crises, doctors become stressed. The hospital doctor reacts by referring to another specialist, and then another specialist, and another and another, until finally the patient goes back to the GP. Good GPs learn to cope sympathetically with such heartsink patients; bad ones burn out.

But the patients can help; by being *patient*; by being understanding; above all else, by having a realistic idea of what a doctor can and cannot achieve.

Personal Hygiene

Grandma always told you to make sure you were wearing clean knickers in case you were knocked over in a road traffic accident and had to go to hospital. Sound advice.

Doctors may be more exposed to bodily fluids, and other human produce of varying vintages, but they do not like it any more than anyone else. Patients think the worst thing doctors have to do is examine genitals and rectums. It is not true. There is nothing wrong with down-to-earth, honest-to-goodness, excrement. There are two things that doctors find much more objectionable:

➢ Examining sweaty and unwashed armpits

➢ Examining the sweaty and unwashed underside of large, pendulous breasts, particularly if as well as not washing the patient has applied layers of talcum powder to produce a stuck on, odoriferous, glutinous mulch.

Both these problems can be avoided by washing.

Journalists

The medical profession is under more media scrutiny than any other profession or occupation. Every day there are documentaries or dramas or both on radio and television . All newspapers have a medical section or medical page, and most of them have a tame media doctor who makes his living criticising the profession to which he used to belong.

It's a free country. We have a free press. No doctor wants to prevent or restrict serious analysis of the medical profession. But there is a problem when 'medical' journalists, who at best can only be partially-informed about current medical theory and practice, shoot from the hip at soft targets without regard for the consequences.

Think of the medical journalist as a cheese sampler. The checsc sampler inserts a long metal tube into the centre of a cheese about which he has no empirical knowledge, and removes a specimen for tasting. Rather like taking a biopsy. When he has tasted his specimen he knows a great deal about a small area in the centre of the cheese.

The medical journalist similarly sticks his probe into the middle of medicine and pulls out a gobbitt of information which he studies intensely. But he knows nothing of the rest of the medical cheese and does not realise that the small specimen he has selected at random is not representative of the whole batch. Still, he reaches four firm conclusions:

• That he is a world expert on the topic.

•That because *he* did not know about the topic before, very few doctors know about it now. Certainly not the GPs, probably not the rest of the British medical profession; but perhaps some experts in the USA.

• That the disease presents a threat to life in Britain, to no small extent because of medical ignorance.

• That it is his duty to educate both the people and the doctors

It becomes his mission in life to 'inform' the country.

Take *Necrotising Fasciitis.*[1] This genuinely dangerous and unpleasant condition is as rare as hens' teeth. It is difficult to treat. It is well known to the medical profession. People sometimes die of it. But only a handful a year. In the same year that half a dozen die of the condition, hundreds will die of paracetamol overdoses because they did not understand that this over-the-counter drug is dangerous, and thousands more will die of tobacco-related diseases. The journalists really could do something to help.

Why don't we get front page articles on "Paracetamol - the drug that eats your liver" or "Tobacco - the hobby that kills"? Because it's old hat

---

[1] Pronounced 'fash-i-itis'

and wouldn't sell papers.

But *Necrotising Fasciitis*, that's something else. It sounds nasty, like something you might catch off a lavatory seat, or from shaking hands with gravediggers. There is just a hint of kinkiness, with that *necro* prefix; never mind that necro is just a foreign word for dead. It has . . . connotations. And, of course, the condition is a **proven killer** – admittedly in such small numbers as to make the risk infinitesimal – but a killer nonetheless.

The newspapers seize on it as a vehicle for sensationalist scaremongering. Implementing the tried-and-tested media formula, they:

1. Frighten the life out of the punter by suggesting that the country is on the cusp of a new bubonic plague;

2. Discredit the GPs - "Your GP has never heard of this condition. Make sure you go straight to hospital."

3. Discredit the British hospital doctors. "People are dying in Britain, but **experts in New York** say this condition can be cured."

And so droves of terrified patients short-circuit their GP, who has the experience to diagnose the condition and refer it in a way that guarantees the patient will be admitted to hospital and treated properly. Instead, they go to the Casualty Officer at the hospital. He is resplendent in his white coat, but readers of the *ODPH* know that he is that most dangerous of medical beasts: the unsupervised SHO. He misdiagnoses the condition and treats it with an inadequate dose of the wrong anti-biotic. The patient

dies and becomes a cause célebre; the family organises charity whist-drives to raise funds to fly other sufferers to America.

It happened with herpes. It happened with *Necrotising Fasciitis*. It will happen again.

Helpful Patients

Imagine you are on a 747 flying from London to New York. Over the Atlantic there is a lot of turbulence and the plane is buffeted. Your son has 'The I-Spy Pop-up Book of Flying' with him. It contains an exploded three dimensional plan of a large plane, with information about how to trim the controls in a storm. You tell the stewardess who immediately takes you up to the cockpit. The pilot is enormously grateful. He asks if he can borrow the book, and suggests you sit in the co-pilot's seat to advise for the rest of the flight.

Alternatively, perhaps you are being prosecuted for a serious criminal offence. Despite legal aid and the best QC in the land to defend you, things do not seem to be going well. Fortunately, you have brought with you the 'Teach Yourself Legal Defence' book, Volumes I and II. You underline a selection of helpful paragraphs in both books and pass them to your barrister. Based on your advice, he is able to modify his whole strategy and you are acquitted. He is immensely grateful and after the trial offers you a job in his Chambers.

If you have had this sort of

experience in a plane or in court, then you must not deprive your doctors of similar help. In particular, they will like:

• to see articles pointing out the many things they did not learn at medical school

• details of the better treatment available for your condition in the USA

• a reading list of medical articles with which you think they should be familiar

• advice on the drugs they should prescribe

If you have yet to advise a professional in this manner, start with a pilot. Consider his reaction carefully, and be guided by it the next time you feel the need to help your doctor.

Symptom Inflation

"Ye can call it influenza if ye like,' said Mrs Machin. 'There was no influenza in my young days. We called a cold a cold."

ARNOLD BENNETT (1867-1931)

A certain kind of patient is unable to describe bodily function without lapsing into hyperbole. He sits in front of the doctor with a smile on his face saying he has been in **"agony"** for two days. All doctors have seen patients with kidney stones, or renal colic. They are in agony. They do not smile. They roll round the floor, screaming.

Children no longer vomit, they **"pump"**. Sweat **"pours"**. Diarrhoea comes in "**torrents**". Adults with headaches are unable to look at bright lights. Children with headaches all have neck stiffness.

Lots of patients suffer from "Unt-hiers" syndrome. They collapse in the chair in front of the doctor and say, "I'm very well really doctor, and would not have bothered you, but I have got pain here *and here and here and here* . . .". It's their third consultation that month, and the seventy-third that year. On average, they come twice a week. Their symptoms are inexplicable, untreatable and entirely compatible with a long life.

If it is not pain everywhere, it is, "I don't know, doctor, I just feel tired all the time." T.A.T.T.-syndrome consumes a vast amount of investigative resources and yields little organic pathology.

Some patients spend ten minutes giving a detailed description of the onset, development and continuance of the common cold. They look with dismay and disbelief at the doctor when he suggests rest and aspirin. They know there is 'proper' treatment for their condition. The doctor has the cure; he just will not give it to them. He is part of a medical conspiracy to deny them relief from illness; to prolong their suffering. They shout and become abusive; they storm out into the waiting room saying it's a waste of time seeing "that" doctor. To get revenge, they call him out that night, forcing him to visit against his better judgement by saying they think they have got pneumonia. He still does not prescribe an antibiotic, so they complain to the FHSA. The complaint is thrown out, but it takes eight months to be processed. Eight months of stress for the doctor. This sort of patient changes doctor frequently until he finds one who doles out antibiotics on request; anything for a quiet life. They deserve each other.

Twenty Ways to Drive Your Doctor Insane

1. Turn up late for an appointment and tell the doctor that you were allowing for the fact that he is always running late.

2. Call doctors who are not surgeons "Mr".

3. Say "I won't keep you, doctor, I've just popped in for an antibiotic."

4. Bring an article from a newspaper suggesting a better treatment for your condition.

5. Ask for something to "throw off" a cold.

6. Bring a diary listing the frequency, form and content of your bowel actions over the last four weeks.

7. Save up a long list of problems for one consultation.

8. Start consultations by saying, "I'm not a tablet person, but..."

9. After listening to your doctor's advice, say "Yes, but I think I'd better have a letter to see someone."

10. Fail to wash your armpits.

11. Try to persuade the doctor to do a home visit by saying that you "pay his bloody wages".

12. When given a prescription, always ask if the medicine is "a drug".

13. Make any reference to the Citizens Charter.

14. Try to help the doctor by diagnosing your own condition.

15. Ask for some treatment that your neighbour's niece, who is a nurse, has recommended.

16. Tell the doctor that little Jason has always been hyperactive, as he smashes up the consulting room.

17. If the doctor declines to give an antibiotic, remind him that his predecessor always used to.

18. Tell the receptionist that if you cannot have an immediate appointment you will go home and call the doctor out.

19. Say you do not know why you are fat because you "do not eat a thing".

20. Tell him how they treat your condition in America.

MEDICAL ETHICS

The GMC

The arbiter of medical ethics in the UK is the General Medical Council (GMC), and all doctors must be registered with it. If a doctor is in breach of medical ethics, he may be reprimanded, suspended from, or even struck off the medical register altogether, thus depriving him of his livelihood.

The public is often outraged that more doctors are not struck off for making mistakes. This is a misunderstanding of the primary function of the GMC. It is not a civil law court, although it does exercise its functions in a judicial fashion. It is not a forum for a victim of medical negligence. It receives many letters a year from people alleging negligence, and will usually suggest they take independent legal advice. That is not to say that doctors who are grossly negligent are not struck off the register sometimes. They may be. But the negligence but first be proved.

The GMC disciplinary committee looks at the behaviour of doctors who are alleged to have behaved *improperly* or *unethically*. Such behaviour may or may not include negligence. The committee will certainly investigate persistent negligence, and negligence that is gross and wilful.

It is a cliché to say that doctors are much more likely to be struck off the register for indecency or improper sexual relations with the patient than for negligently mistreating them. It is a cliché because, like all clichés, it is true.

Sleeping with the Enemy

"Never believe what a patient tells you his doctor said."

SIR WILLIAM JENNER (1815-98)

Doctors are allowed to sleep with their patients.

There! You didn't know that did you? But they are. It is not illegal. It is not unethical. You can sleep with your architect. You can sleep with your accountant. You can sleep with your bank manager. And many people do. So why deprive yourself of a little medical nookey?

The question that concerns the GMC is whether the doctor has used his professional position to influence the patient unduly in her decision to sleep with him. Has he abused the doctor-patient relationship?

If a doctor sleeps with a patient who is married to someone else, and the cuckolded partner complains, there may be an evidential assumption that the doctor-patient relationship has been so abused, and the doctor will have to prove his "innocence." The lawyers have a Latin phrase for this. *Res ipsa loquitur*: "the thing speaks for itself."

If a fifty-seven year old edentulous gynaecologist has got himself into a leg-over situation with a sixteen-year old girl who he happens to be treating for dysmenorrhoea, there will be an evidential assumption of guilt and undue influence. We do not need a pretentious Latin phrase to realise that there has been a bit of hanky-panky going on and that the gynaecologist has some explaining to do. But lawyers have a Latin phrase for everything; it helps to justify their fees.

Wine, Women and Song

"If you want to keep a dead man, put him in whiskey; if you want to kill a live man put whiskey in him."

THOMAS GUTHRIE (1803-73)

Wine, women and song is a misleading sub-heading. The GMC does not disapprove of song, and many of the finest rugby songs have been composed and are regularly sung by doctors. Women have already been covered, so to speak, and so that just leaves wine. And whiskey. And gin. And beer. And rum. And brandy. And methylated spirits.

It is rumoured that some doctors drink too much. This is not true. A lot of doctors drink too much.

The reasons for this are well known to readers of the *ODPH*. It is part of medical machismo. It is part of medical training. It is a human reaction to long hours and the stress of dealing every day with pain and suffering. But if these factors go towards explanation and even mitigation, they do not provide a justification.

The GMC disapproves strongly of alcohol-related problems and says:

"...convictions for drunkenness or other offences arising from the misuse of alcohol (such as driving under the influence of alcohol) indicate habits which are discreditable to the profession and may be a source of danger to the doctor's patients."

In 1991 the preliminary proceedings committee of the GMC received notice of twenty-eight doctors who had been convicted of alcohol abuse and two convicted of failure to provide a breath specimen. These notifications resulted in seventeen letters of admonishment and eleven adjournments *sine die* for health procedures - in other words, "Get a doctor, doctor". No doctors were struck off the register for drunkenness.

So alcohol and doctors do not seem to represent a big threat to patients. But do not be misled. There is an enormous threat to patients; a threat that originates in medical hypocrisy: Because

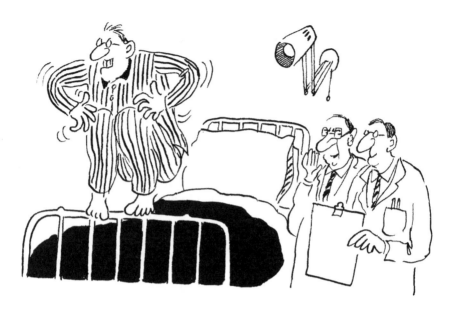

" . . and if anyone asks where we got the heart, just don't mention Regent's Park."

doctors are so self-conscious about the bad example their own profession sets, they are quick to condemn any sign of alcohol excess in others.

Never, ever, go to a doctor smelling of alcohol

Even if you only drink one glass of white wine a year, on your birthday, if you see the doctor on that day, there will be an entry in your medical notes saying "Smelt strongly of alcohol at..." and a time will be entered. Doctors are particularly unimpressed if the time is deemed to be inappropriate. The definition of 'inappropriate' is arbitrary but tied to pub opening hours. As doctors for some reason do not have surgeries when pubs are open, the time will usually be deemed to be inappropriate.

When the doctor asks you how much you drink never say "Just an occasional glass of white wine". Doctors regard this as the quintessential understatement of the alcoholic. The remark will be entered in your notes, probably in red, with inverted commas round it and three exclamation remarks after it. You would be better advised to admit to three flagons of cider and a quart of methylated spirits a day. This at least has the merit of sounding truthful to the alcohol obsessed doctor.

Once there is any suggestion in your medical notes that you have an alcohol problem it will be passed from doctor to doctor and will prejudice each and every one of them against you. It will be quoted to insurance companies when you have to provide medical evidence of health. It will be quoted to prospective employers if you need a medical reference for a job.

Doctors love to chastise patients. It used to be smoking but so many have stopped smoking that alcohol has taken over.

The 'Gold Standard' of safe alcohol intake was set in 1987 at fourteen units per week for women and twenty-one units a week for men. The medical profession is at present incredulous and embarrassed, as it is emerging that not only might these levels have been set far too low but that a higher intake may actually promote health and prolong life.

This raises the fascinating possibility that those millions of patients who have derogatory remarks in their medical notes about problem drinking may be able to sue their doctors for defamation. Just wait until lawyers find out.

Getting Struck Off

It does not happen very often.

The procedure followed by the GMC is thorough and judicial. All complaints are carefully considered by a preliminary screening committee. Most will be dealt with informally, often by advising the complainant that they need to take their grievance elsewhere. When there is evidence of serious professional misconduct, the case is referred to the Professional Conduct Committee.

A thorough investigation is held. There may be a full hearing at which both the GMC and the accused doctor are entitled to legal representation.

As the doctor's career may be at stake, the lawyers will be leading counsel.

In 1990 a total of fifty-five cases were considered; thirteen doctors were struck off, ten were suspended, thirteen were admonished, six were given conditional registration (i.e. could only continue working under supervision); three were referred to the health committee and nine were found not guilty. One case was adjourned. In 1992, forty-four cases were considered and fourteen doctors were struck off.

The reasons given for depriving doctors of their right to practise appear in the table over the page. They sound bland and unexciting but don't be fooled; they cover some horrific abuses:

'Irregularities relating to Surgical Operations' in this instance referred to the buying and selling of organs for transplant, often without the donors' informed consent.

'False Claims concerning Treatment' referred to two doctors who fleeced HIV victims by purporting to sell a cure.

'False Returns to a Drug Company' concerned a doctor who was paid a fee to do research, who did not do the research, but submitted results, which were entirely bogus.

If buying and selling human organs without the donors informed consent constitutes 'irregularities' the mind boggles as to what indecency might include.

SUMMARY OF REASONS FOR . . . . STRIKING OFF

	1990	1992
Disregard of professional responsibilities to patients	2	4
Indecency	5	3
Improper prescribing or supplying of drugs	1	0
Dishonesty	1	0
Improper relationship with patients	2	0
Irregularities in relation to surgical operations	1	0
False claims to professional qualifications	1	0
Providing treatment for which not qualified or trained	0	2
False claims concerning treatment	0	2
False returns to drug companies in connection with drug trials	0	1
TOTALS	**13**	**12**

SUING A DOCTOR

The patient died so the doctor must have been negligent

"Early to rise and early to bed
Makes a male healthy, wealthy
and dead"

JAMES THURBER (1894-1961)

In the United States, death is an avoidable event provided you eat margarine, drink spritzers and jog regularly. It follows that if a patient dies, or fails to make a complete recovery from a serious illness, the doctor must have made a mistake and should be sued.

Medico-legal litigation in the USA is so prevalent that many doctors in the high-risk specialities have difficulty affording the negligence insurance premiums despite the large incomes they earn. It can be hard to find a doctor prepared, for example, to deliver a baby. The Caesarean section rate has risen to over a quarter of all deliveries because of doctors' anxieties about the dangers of normal childbirth. Madwives are not allowed to conduct deliveries at all, which is a mistake. No one would dare sue a madwife.

Because of the huge awards being made in negligence cases, doctors in the US now practise medicine looking over their shoulders at the lawyers behind them. They practise 'defensive medicine'.

Defensive Medicine

Doctors in the US perform investigations not necessarily in the patients' best interests, but so that, should the need arise, they can demonstrate to the judge and jury that no stone was left unturned.

The concept of defensive medicine is fatally flawed. In a famous medico-legal case in Britain, *Whitehouse v Jordan*, a baby sustained brain damage during a prolonged attempt to effect a forceps delivery. The question was whether the obstetrician had pulled too long and too hard on the forceps before proceeding to an emergency Caesarean Section. It was finally decided that he had not been negligent. One of the appeal court judges said defensive medicine consists of:

"...adopting procedures which are not for the benefit of the patient but safeguard against the possibility of the patient making a claim for negligence."

208

It follows that *positive* defensive medicine involves subjecting patients to investigations that are not necessary on medical grounds alone. If they are not necessary, they should not be done. If they should not be done and they are done, the patient may succeed in a claim for unnecessary pain and suffering. The British courts, unlike the American, have robustly supported this position.

Not having to practise defensive medicine of course does not allow the British doctor to be cavalier. There is still no room for cock-ups. The classic cock-up, for which doctors are sued every year, is leaving something in at the operation. Something that should not be left in; something that is additional to normal bodily requirements; something like swabs, forceps and the surgeon's contact lenses. Patients whinge terribly when they find that a bit of surgical ironmongery is cluttering up their abdominal cavity. It's best not to tell them if possible. It rarely does them any harm. Out of sight, out of mind. Patients think it does not happen very often. Why disabuse them of this comforting feeling?

A survey of twenty crematoria in Greater London carried out in 1993 [1] showed a wide variety of unexpected metal residues found amongst the ashes of the recently departed. These included Spencer Wells forceps, Jean's forceps, Artery forceps, a pacemaker, a ring cutter and a pair of Mayo scissors.

And these were patients who did not sue.

[1] Barry M. 'Metal residues after cremation' BMJ 1994, 308-390

The Defence Organisations

The majority of doctors in this country are members of a medical defence organisation. The two best known ones are The Medical Defence Union (MDU) and the Medical Protection Society (MPS). They act like specialist insurance companies (technically they are not insurance companies) and are staffed by medico-legally trained doctors.

The annual subscription for doctors is between one and two thousand pounds per year. It varies very slightly between the organisations and depends upon which speciality the doctor is in.

This premium provides unlimited liability for negligence claims including all damages and legal costs. There is no limit to the number of claims that can be made and members with a 'bad record' are not thrown out.

Doctors often moan about the cost of this insurance. Few realise that it is the envy of all other professionals who pay much higher indemnity premiums and even then can rarely purchase cover for unlimited liability.

It used to be a condition of hospital jobs that all doctors should be members of a recognised defence union. This requirement has now been dropped as doctors in the hospital service are covered by Crown Immunity. The wise ones have continued their membership of a defence union for reasons that will become clear.

Provided he is a member of a defence union, the doctor who is being sued gets the best legal advice in the country at no cost to himself.

The Plaintiff

The litigious layman assumes that very high damages will be awarded against a doctor who has, for example, just murdered his – the plaintiff's – grandmother. This is not so. A small amount may be recovered for grief and suffering and certainly something to cover funeral expenses, but that will be it. There will be no telephone number awards as are seen in the USA.

Good legal advice is essential. Suing for revenge, or to make an example of a doctor, is an expensive undertaking with no guarantee of financial return. Even if you win, the defendant may not have to pay all your legal bills, which can easily eclipse any compensation you receive.

Solicitors who specialise in medical negligence will charge a hundred and twenty pounds an hour upwards, and at the blue-chip City of London firms it may be up to three times that rate. On top of that there will be fees for medical experts and barristers.

The doctor, meanwhile, has a powerful and sophisticated organisation behind him, which devotes all its time to defending doctors accused of negligence. There is no comparable organisation for the plaintiff.

The Legal Lottery

The Royal Commission on Civil Liability and Compensation for Personal Injury (1978) reported on the likelihood of plaintiffs succeeding in actions for negligence. Eighty-five per cent of all plaintiffs are successful whereas only thirty to forty per cent of plaintiffs suing for medical negligence succeed. More recent evidence suggests that the success rate in medical negligence actions has fallen during the 1980's to approximately twenty-five per cent.

Why should this be? Have the MDU and MPS got doctors so well protected that they can get away with murder? Literally? This is only part of the story.

Certainly, the defence organisations are formidably effective. But they are also reputable and are not in the business of unjustly or unfairly depriving patients of compensation for negligence.

Defending Doctors

When a doctor is sued for negligence, his defence union will consider all the facts of the case and take advice from eminent medical experts as to whether the doctor can reasonably be defended. If the conclusion is that he has been negligent, immediate attempts will be made to settle the case out of court with the payment of appropriate damages. The case will come to court only if the plaintiff is not prepared to accept the damages offered.

If, on the other hand, the defence union concludes that the doctor has not been negligent and has a reasonable defence, they will not settle. However long it takes, and whatever the cost, the doctor will be defended and every effort made to keep his reputation untarnished.

And this is why the statistics show so few plaintiffs succeeding. The majority of cases in which there is merit in the action are settled out of court with an appropriate payment of damages.

The hospital doctors who decide to save a few pounds a week by not joining a defence union lose out. A hospital does not carry negligence insurance and bears its own costs. Its sole interest is to save money and saving money often means settling out of court even though there is no merit in the complaint. In other words, a vexatious but determined litigant is bought off. The question of the doctor's reputation is secondary.

There is a further problem. Hospital administrators tend to deal with complaints personally without taking legal advice. They inflame the complainants by being obstructive; by refusing to confirm simple and obvious facts which lawyers would soon agree as common ground; by prevaricating about the patient's right to see his notes; and worst of all, by refusing to offer an apology. This is foolish. The facts will emerge eventually. And sooner rather than later. Refusing to hand over notes only aggravates the situation. Leaving apart any question of statutory requirements, well before a court case commences there is a system of discovery of documents where each side must reveal to the other pertinent documents upon which they intend to rely. Finally and if necessary, the court will order the hospital to produce the notes and the trial judge will take a dim view of any prevarication.

Barrack room lawyers assume that any form of apology is an admission of full liability and is therefore to be avoided. Hospital administrators are for ever refusing to apologise.

Most victims of medical accidents, even when there has been negligence, do not set out looking for damages and compensation. Three months argument with a stroppy and autocratic hospital administrator forces reluctant plaintiffs into court. Often all they want is a clear and comprehensive explanation as to what went wrong and a sympathetic hearing of their point of view. A gracious apology, when appropriate, may stop a complaint in its tracks even when there has been gross and obvious negligence.

Apologies may hurt but they are cheaper than lawyers.

Also published by Harriman House

'The Official
Lawyer's Handbook'

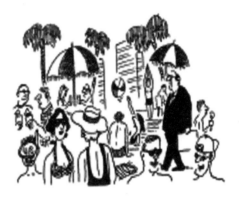

Can you spot the lawyer ?

"One of the most irreverent, funny, and perceptive books about the legal profession has just been published."   *The Times*

"The *Spitting Image* of the legal world: irreverent, biting, and often in delightfully questionable taste."   *The Lawyer*

" . . . . combines a litany of barbed quips with sound advice."
The Law Society Gazette

"A jokey guide to the sleazy world of the solicitor, full of sage advice."   *The Independent on Sunday*

ISBN 1897597002 £8.99. Credit card order 01730 233870 for 24-hr delivery